400 CALORIE FIX TRACKER

Keep Track of Your Favorite Fixes!

RODALE

By Liz Vaccariello Editor-in-Chief of **Prevention**

Photos on pages i, 1, 4, 7, 16, 18–209 (even-numbered journal pages), 211 (center), 213 (top), 214 (top), 218 (top), and 220 (bottom) © Ted Morrison; photo on page 217 (bottom) © John Hamel; photos on page 9, 210, 211 (top & bottom), 212, 213 (center & bottom), 214 (center & bottom), 215, 216, 217 (top & center), 218 (center & bottom), 219, and 220 (top & center) © Mitch Mandel/Rodale Images.

Book design by Jill Armus

Library of Congress Cataloging-in-Publication Data

400 calorie health tracker / Liz Vaccariello, editor-in-chief, with Mindy Hermann.
    p.   cm.
  ISBN-13 978–1–60529–532–9 pbk.
  ISBN-10 1–60529–532–9 pbk.
  1. Reducing diets. 2. Exercise. 3. Account books. I. Vaccariello, Liz. II. Hermann, Mindy G. III. Title: Four hundred calorie health tracker.
RM222.2.F678 2010
613.2'3—dc22   2009043877

2 4 6 8 10 9 7 5 3 1   paperback

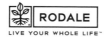

RODALE
LIVE YOUR WHOLE LIFE™

We inspire and enable people to improve their lives and the world around them

For more of our products visit **rodalestore.com** or call 800-848-4735

Introduction

Year after year, diet after diet, you've reduced your fat intake, made your meals low-carb, and tried every sugar substitute you could find. But you're still putting on an extra 2 or 4 or 10 pounds a year. What's the problem? The research is clear. Experts say that food, and too much of it, is the reason why the United States is now in the midst of an obesity epidemic. According to the US Department of Agriculture (USDA) Economic Research Service, the average American ate about 2,200 calories per day in 1970. By 2007, that was up to 2,800 calories per day.

Most of us don't know how many calories are in the foods we eat. And most of us don't really want to have to count calories. Moreover, only 15 percent of adults know how many calories a person of their age, height, and activity level should eat to maintain a healthy weight—the rest either estimate incorrectly or are totally unaware—and most of us aren't even entirely sure what our healthy weight should be![1]

Research shows that most people underestimate portions and

---

[1] International Food Information Council. 2009 Food & Health Survey: Consumer Attitudes toward Food, Nutrition & Health. www.ific.org

calories. In one study, 120 men and women selected premeasured foods from a buffet line and then told the research team how much food they thought they had eaten. Less than one-third was able to estimate portions correctly.[2] In another survey, respondents who were asked to estimate the calories and fat in nine restaurant entrées generally were off by 100 percent—they thought that a meal with more than 1,300 calories had only 642 calories.[3]

So what's the fix? Too much food may be the problem, but as someone with a deep appreciation for the power of food to heal, fuel, and energize, I know that food can also be part of the solution. And now, as editor-in-chief of *Prevention* magazine and coauthor of the blockbuster *Flat Belly Diet!*, I see a clear, simple, back-to-basics trend emerging: It all comes down to calories.

The latest scientific studies are backing up calorie control as the smartest means of achieving a healthy weight and a long life. Yes, it's just that simple: The only way to lose weight and keep it off long-term is to learn how to spot and control calories. Here's some of the recent research that got me excited.

✤ Several studies on calorie control were linked to better sensitivity to insulin and, potentially, to longer life in humans.[4]

✤ More than 800 overweight adults who were assigned to one of four lower-calorie diets—low fat, high carb; low fat, moderate carb;

---

[2] California Center for Public Health Advocacy. March 20–31, 2007, statewide poll. (http://www.publichealthadvocacy.org/menulabelingpoll.html)

[3] Burton S, et al. "Attacking the obesity epidemic: the potential health benefits of providing nutrition information in restaurants." *Am J Public Health*. 2006; 96: 1669–75.

[4] Redman LM, Ravussin E. "Endocrine alterations in response to calorie restriction in humans." *Mol Cell Endocrinol*. 2009 Feb 5; 299(1): 129–36. Epub 2008 Oct 21.

high fat, low carb; and high fat, very low carb—lost about the same amount of weight over 2 years, *regardless of which diet they were on.*[5]
♣ Blood pressure, fasting blood glucose, insulin levels, and resistance to insulin all decreased in a group of adults who were on a 1-year, calorie-controlled weight loss diet.[6]

Inspired by this simple idea—control calories to control your weight—I enlisted the help of Mindy Hermann, RD, a prominent registered dietitian and food expert, to create the 400 Calorie Fix. This is a flexible, easy-to-follow eating plan that controls calories but also allows for splurges and favorite foods. And to help you make the best use of this powerful lifestyle fix, we put together the food and activity tracker you hold in your hands to keep you motivated and inspired!

---

[5] Sacks FM et al. "Comparison of weight-loss diets with different compositions of fat, protein, and carbohydrates." *N Engl J Med.* 2009; 360: 859–73.
[6] Brinkworth GD et al. "Long-term effects of a very-low-carbohydrate weight loss diet compared with an isocaloric low-fat diet after 12 mo." *Am J Clin Nutr.* 2009 May 13. [Epub ahead of print]

The MAGIC NUMBER

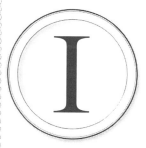

IF YOU'RE A WOMAN of average size and average activity level, you need about 1,600 calories per day to maintain a healthy weight (that's four 400-calorie meals a day). But when it comes to weight and calories, one size does not fit all. According to government estimates, most men need about 2,000 calories a day; hence, the use of a 2,000-calorie standard on food package labels. Athletes and other people who are very active may need more. But if you're trying to lose weight rather than maintain your current weight, you probably need less.

Regardless of our total calorie needs, though, we all need food to fuel us throughout our busy day. Skipping breakfast, having a light lunch, and then eating a really big dinner (which many of us do) doesn't meet the body's daylong need for calories and nutrients. Eating 1,600 calories a day that way—that is, almost all in one meal—is a recipe for moodiness and exhaustion. You'll be hungry and suffer from low blood sugar during the day, *plus* your body won't metabolize fat as efficiently, especially at night.

Study after study recommends spacing out your meals at regular intervals and keeping them all about the same size. Irregular meals have been linked to fewer calories burned after eating, better response to insulin, and lower fasting blood cholesterol levels. When you eat regular meals throughout the day, you're less likely to become ravenous and to overeat. You also keep your blood sugar levels balanced, your metabolism revved, and your mood stable.

Historically, some calorie-controlled diets were hard to follow because they didn't take hunger into account—or what the best types of foods were to keep energy levels up and cravings at bay. Mindy and I chose 400 calories as our per-meal "fix" because it's the right amount to keep you active and satiated until your next meal. Plus it allows for variety—go any lower, and it would be difficult to get a good mix of tastes and textures on your plate, as well as enough body-building, disease-fighting nutrients.

Here's how it works: Each of the 400-plus meals in the *400 Calorie Fix* delivers between 380 and 420 calories. You will eat three, four, or five meals a day, depending on your gender and activity level (and how much weight you want to lose). So if you choose three meals daily, you'll get about 1,200 calories; four daily meals provide about 1,600 calories; and five daily meals serve up 2,000 calories.

Just consult the chart below to determine the number of meals you should eat per day (and your daily calorie count).

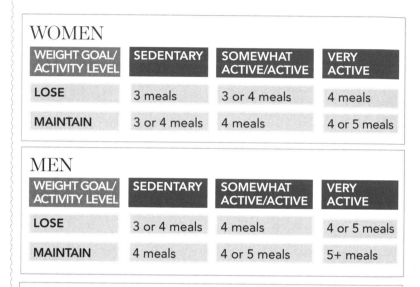

WOMEN

WEIGHT GOAL/ ACTIVITY LEVEL	SEDENTARY	SOMEWHAT ACTIVE/ACTIVE	VERY ACTIVE
LOSE	3 meals	3 or 4 meals	4 meals
MAINTAIN	3 or 4 meals	4 meals	4 or 5 meals

MEN

WEIGHT GOAL/ ACTIVITY LEVEL	SEDENTARY	SOMEWHAT ACTIVE/ACTIVE	VERY ACTIVE
LOSE	3 or 4 meals	4 meals	4 or 5 meals
MAINTAIN	4 meals	4 or 5 meals	5+ meals

SEDENTARY—You sit most of the day and drive everywhere, and you log in plenty of hours of screen time each day.

SOMEWHAT ACTIVE—You get about 30 minutes of physical activity daily. Nothing too strenuous, generally the equivalent of walking about $1\frac{1}{2}$ to 3 miles daily, or 3,000 to 6,000 steps on a pedometer.

ACTIVE—You like to move around and you clock 30 to 60 minutes of daily physical activity by climbing stairs at the office, parking farther away at the market, plus moderate exercise (the equivalent of walking more than 3 miles per day, or more than 6,000 steps on a pedometer).

VERY ACTIVE—You're more than a weekend warrior; you thrive on high intensity sports and rigorous activities that total more than 60 minutes per day.

The
TOOLS

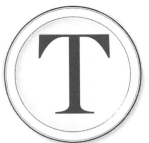

T HE *400 CALORIE FIX* gives you an important gift—a set of powerful tools to help you see your meals through a 400 Calorie Lens no matter what you like to eat or where you are. You decide which tools are best for you. Each on its own puts you on the path to more healthful eating the 400-calorie way. But they all are designed to work together to create a powerful weight loss solution.

Now, with the *400 Calorie Fix Tracker*, we've created yet another valuable tool to help you take charge of your eating, your weight, and your health. The tracker is designed to work primarily with two of the most effective components in the tool kit.

❖ **THE 400 CALORIE LENS**—visual tricks and shortcuts for selecting foods that add up to 400 calories, wherever you eat.

❖ **THE 4 STAR NUTRITION SYSTEM**—your guide to nutritional balance, with meals starred based on their fruits and vegetables, fiber, protein foods, and healthful fats.

The 400 Calorie Lens

Why are portions, and the calories in them, so hard for us to gauge? Because an appropriate portion of food varies, depending on the type of food and the way it's prepared. Pound for pound, nuts pack more calories than apples, apples more than lettuce, lettuce dipped in creamy salad dressing more than plain lettuce, and so on. Because there are multiple factors that affect your food portions, we've given you multiple options for calculating portions and calories. Use as many as you find helpful.

❖ **WEIGH AND MEASURE**—It can be tedious, but it's the most accurate way to tell how much food you're eating. Invest in a set of measuring cups and spoons and a food scale.

❖ **SEE THE VISUAL CUES**—When you're eating away from home and don't have access to your measuring tools, use visual cues to eyeball, say, a steak or a bowl of pasta and have a reasonably good idea of how big or small it is (see the chart at right). The *400 Calorie Fix* gives you a choice of two sets of visual shortcuts, one using your hand as a reference, the other using a series of balls of different sizes.

❖ **KNOW YOUR COMMON FOODS**—While of course you can't memorize all the foods in the world and their calorie counts, you'll probably get to know the right portions of your favorite foods over time. The list of foods in the back of this book gives you some common foods to start with.

❖ **LEARN THE "1-2-3-400-CALORIE TRICK"**—Once you have an idea of the appropriate portions for individual foods, it's time to put them together to make balanced meals. So we came up with a quick system to give you the right balance of nutrients while staying in the 400-calorie ballpark.

(continued on page 10)

It's a ball, it's a hand, it's a portion

	BALL	HAND	PORTIONS	EXAMPLES
	Small marble	Tip of the thumb	1 teaspoon	oil, butter, margarine, sugar
	Large marble	Base of thumb to first knuckle	1 table-spoon	chopped nuts, honey, ketchup
	Two large marbles	Whole thumb	2 table-spoons/ 1 ounce liquid	salad dressing, grated cheese, raisins, sliced olives, guacamole
	Golf ball	Cupped handful	¼ cup	beans, chopped vegetables, salsa, hummus
	Hockey puck	Palm of the hand	½ cup/ 4 oz (¼ lb) raw meat, poultry, fish	burger patty, sliced deli meat, beef, pork, chicken, turkey, fish
	Tennis ball	Open handful	½ cup	rice, pasta, fruit salad, melon balls, small roll, scrambled eggs
	Wiffle ball	Very loose cupped handful	1 cup/ 1 to 2 ounces chips	potato chips, tortilla chips, popcorn, pretzels
	Baseball	Whole fist	1 cup	cereal, lettuce, vegetables, strawberries, soup

Divide your plate into six sections.

- Fill **one** section with one serving of a protein. For meat, chicken, or fish, that's 3 ounces cooked, about the size of a hockey puck. One cup of milk or yogurt also provides one serving of protein.
- Fill **two** sections with two servings of a grain food like rice, pasta, or bread. For rice and pasta, that's ²/₃ cup, or slightly less than a baseball-size scoop of rice or pasta. For bread, it's two slices (no butter, though!).
- Fill **three** sections with three servings of vegetables. Each serving is 1 cup, so pile on three baseball-size heaps of greens and other veggies.

✤ **SPY HIDDEN CALORIES**—Fats and sugars can add a lot of calories in very small, tasty packages, so be vigilant about spotting them.

The 4 Star Nutrition System

The 4 Star Nutrition System will help you eat for health *and* nutrition while following a 400-calorie lifestyle. To create the 4 Star System, Mindy identified four important features in healthy meals: protein, good fats, fiber, and fruits and vegetables. We then assigned each a star and determined a threshold for each feature, awarding stars accordingly. Some of the meals have just one star. Others have two, three, even four stars because they qualify in more than one category. A few meals have zero stars. These are our Fun Meals, like ice cream, cake, and ballpark food, which fall short of our nutrition guidelines but still have a place in a healthy (real) life.

Mindy designed each of the 400+ meals in the *400 Calorie Fix* book to be as nutritionally balanced as possible. Almost all of the meals— even some of our Fun Meals—include more than one of these four key elements. (In other words, just because a meal doesn't have a good fats star doesn't mean it doesn't have any good fats in it; it just doesn't have quite enough to qualify for that star.) Because it is virtually impossible to get enough of all four components in just one meal, it's more important to look at the balance of protein, good fats, fiber, and fruits and vegetables over the course of a day. Here's a closer look at these essential foods and nutrients.

✤ **PROTEIN STAR, AT LEAST 20 GRAMS PER MEAL**—We get most of our protein from meats, poultry, fish, seafood, eggs, and dairy products, along with plant-based sources such as legumes (kidney and other dried beans, split peas and other kinds of peas, and lentils), soy, and nuts. When eating meat, choose lean cuts, and take the skin off poultry to reduce the amount of fat, saturated fat, and calories you consume. Bite for bite, plant sources are a smart choice; while they are not quite as rich in protein, they usually supply fiber and have almost no saturated fat.

✤ **GOOD FATS STAR, AT LEAST ONE FOOD ITEM THAT SUPPLIES A SIGNIFICANT AMOUNT OF MUFA OR OMEGA-3s**—Monounsaturated fatty acids (MUFAs) are found mainly in nuts, olives, olive and canola oils, avocados, and chocolate. Omega-3s are the main fats in fish and other seafood. Like all fats, they are calorie dense, so be especially careful to apply the 400 Calorie Lens to keep your portions in check.

✤ **FIBER STAR, AT LEAST 7 GRAMS PER MEAL**—To increase your fiber intake, focus on whole grains, beans, and fruits and vegetables. Some of these foods can cause gas and discomfort if you're not used to eating them regularly. Products like Beano can help.

✤ **FRUITS AND VEGETABLES STAR, AT LEAST 1 CUP PER MEAL**—The meals marked with the fruits and vegetables star include at least 1 cup of fruit, vegetables, or a combination of the two. You can up the ante by adding even more vegetables from the list of free foods on page 12. You'll notice that the list contains a lot of salad veggies, so if a meal that you like doesn't include a green salad, add one topped with a squeeze of lemon juice, a sprinkle of balsamic vinegar, or a few squirts of 1-calorie-per-squirt salad dressing spray.

FREEBIES

Although freebies are not entirely calorie-free, they are low enough to be free if you enjoy them in reasonable portions. The free veggies and condiments are particularly well suited to sandwiches, burgers, and salads.

RAW VEGGIES
Alfalfa sprouts
Bean sprouts
Broccoli
Cabbage
Celery
Cucumber
Dill pickles
Jalapeño chile peppers
Lettuce
Mushrooms
Peppers
Onions
Sauerkraut
Spinach
Tomato

CONDIMENTS
Capers
Hot pepper sauce
Ketchup*
Lemon juice
Mustard
Prepared horseradish
Tomato-pepper salsas
Soy sauce*
Vinegars
Worcestershire sauce
Reduced- or low-sodium

BEVERAGES
Black coffee or tea with no or noncaloric sweeteners
Diet colas or sports drinks
Sparkling water

Using the 4 Star Nutrition System is as simple as collecting stars. Your goal? To collect at least one of each star by the end of the day. The more stars, the better. That's it. See, I told you it was easy! Don't worry about getting too much of any of these ingredients: Because each meal is portion controlled, you can't go overboard even if you wind up with five of each star in a day. And enjoy a Fun Meal—no stars—up to three times a week to stay happy so you can indulge without overdoing it.

The
FIXES

The Big Fix
EAT 400-CALORIE MEALS.

Remember that 400 calories per meal is our chosen number. It's big enough for plenty of food and variety. It's small enough to help you lose weight. And 400-calorie meals are filling, especially when packed with hunger-quelling foods like fruits and vegetables, protein-rich options, high-fiber choices, and nuts and other healthful fats.

Mini Fix #1
EAT THE RIGHT NUMBER OF MEALS.

Use the chart on page 6 to choose the number of daily meals to eat based on your gender, level of physical activity, and weight goal. If after about 2 weeks you are losing up to 2 pounds each week and are not yet at your goal weight, or if you are holding steady at your goal weight, stick with your current meal pattern. If your weight loss is continuing at a faster clip—especially after the first couple of weeks, when weight loss tends to be fastest—consider adding one more daily meal. And if you're gaining weight, you may need to cut out one meal. But don't go below three meals, or 1,200 calories, a day; eating too few calories can cause your metabolism to slow way down, and it's virtually impossible to meet your body's nutritional needs at that level. Also, before you cut out a meal, be sure to double-check your portion sizes just in case you're dishing up more food than you think.

Mini Fix #2
SPACE MEALS EVENLY THROUGHOUT THE DAY.

Do what you can to eat every 4 or 5 hours. You'll find that you're hungry by mealtime, but not so hungry that it's hard to control your eating and food decisions. Record your mealtimes on the pages in this tracker.

Mini Fix #3
REMAIN VIGILANT ABOUT PORTIONS.

It's important to keep up your portion training in order to stay sharp and on top of your diet. So use at least one of the 400-calorie tools every week or so to double-check whether you are still seeing foods through the 400 Calorie Lens.

Mini Fix #4
SEEK NUTRITION.

Your body needs both the right number of calories and the right amount of nutrition, and the 4 Star Nutrition System is an easy-to-use guide for ensuring that your daily diet provides important nutrients—vitamins and minerals from fruits and vegetables, fiber, protein, and healthful fats. We recommend a minimum of four different stars in a day; more stars mean more nutrition in your day. Use the pages in this tracker to keep tabs on the number of stars you're getting every day.

Mini Fix #5
WEIGH YOURSELF.

Weighing yourself at a regular interval—daily, a few days a week, once a week—helps you see how well you're doing. Getting on that scale really does work. Participants in the National Weight Control Registry, a database of more than 5,000 people who lost at least 30 pounds and kept it off for at least a year, say that they weigh themselves frequently.[7] Again, use the pages in this tracker to monitor your progress.

Mini Fix #6
KEEP A FOOD JOURNAL.

Write down what you eat in this handy tracker. People who monitor themselves by keeping a food journal, along with other measures like weighing, have an easier time managing their weight. In a study conducted at the University of Pennsylvania, 49 participants who kept a daily food log and attended group meetings in addition to taking a weight loss medication lost 27 pounds over the course of a year, while 45 participants on medication alone lost just 11 pounds.[8]

Mini Fix #7
GET MOVING.

The other side of the calorie equation is, of course, about calories burned—and that, primarily, is about exercise and movement. Check out the list at the end of this book to learn how much you can burn through your favorite activity, and record it in the pages of this tracker.

---

[7] Wing RR, Phelan S. "Long-term weight loss maintenance." *Am J Clin Nutr.* 2005 Jul; 82(1 Suppl): 222S–225S.

[8] Wadden TA, Berkowitz RI, Womble LG, et al. "Randomized trial of lifestyle modification and pharmacotherapy for obesity." *N Engl J Med* 2005; 353: 2111–20.

HOW TO USE
THE TRACKER

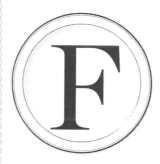

or each day, write the date and your weight. While it's not necessary to weigh yourself every day, it's a good idea to do so at regular intervals (say, once a week) to keep track of your progress. Try to weigh yourself at the same time of day and on the same scale each time.

There is room for you to record up to five meals per day. For each meal, note the time of day and write down what you ate, being as specific as possible. Then mark the total calories for the meal and check off how many stars you collected of each color. You may also find it helpful to observe how hungry you were before and after each meal—we suggest that you use a scale from 1 (starving) to 10 (stuffed) to rate your hunger. Finally, tally up your total calories and total stars for the whole day.

Next, note your activity for the day. Remember to include any physical activity that gets you moving, not just gym trips or long walks.

We've also provided some blank space to record whatever you feel would be helpful to you. You may choose to track other health measurements such as your blood pressure or blood sugar levels (especially if you have or are at risk for diabetes). You may want to note how many hours you've slept, how much energy you have, or whether you still have midafternoon cookie cravings. Or, you may just jot down your favorite foods, observations about when you find it hardest to stick to your plan, or inspirational messages to keep yourself going—whatever is most helpful to you.

Just like the *400 Calorie Fix*, this tracker is designed to be customizable so that you can track what's important to you. It's simple, it's powerful, and it's made just for you. We hope it helps you keep eating the 400-calorie way for life!

date:

weight:

MEAL #1

WHAT I ATE

CALORIES   TIME OF DAY

HUNGER BEFORE   HUNGER AFTER

STARS: ☐ PROTEIN   ☐ FIBER   ☐ GOOD FATS   ☐ FRUITS/VEGGIES

MEAL #2

WHAT I ATE

CALORIES   TIME OF DAY

HUNGER BEFORE   HUNGER AFTER

STARS: ☐ PROTEIN   ☐ FIBER   ☐ GOOD FATS   ☐ FRUITS/VEGGIES

MEAL #3

WHAT I ATE

CALORIES   TIME OF DAY

HUNGER BEFORE   HUNGER AFTER

STARS: ☐ PROTEIN   ☐ FIBER   ☐ GOOD FATS   ☐ FRUITS/VEGGIES

MEAL #4

WHAT I ATE

CALORIES	TIME OF DAY
HUNGER BEFORE	HUNGER AFTER

STARS: ☐ PROTEIN ☐ FIBER ☐ GOOD FATS ☐ FRUITS/VEGGIES

MEAL #5

WHAT I ATE

CALORIES	TIME OF DAY
HUNGER BEFORE	HUNGER AFTER

STARS: ☐ PROTEIN ☐ FIBER ☐ GOOD FATS ☐ FRUITS/VEGGIES

PHYSICAL ACTIVITY

Activity:
Duration:
Intensity:
Calories Burned:

Activity:
Duration:
Intensity:
Calories Burned:

OTHER NOTES

TOTAL CALORIES FOR THE DAY:

TOTAL STARS FOR THE DAY:

Protein
⌐ ⌐ ⌐ ⌐ ⌐
_____

Fiber
⌐ ⌐ ⌐ ⌐ ⌐
_____

Good Fats
⌐ ⌐ ⌐ ⌐ ⌐
_____

Fruits/Veggies
⌐ ⌐ ⌐ ⌐ ⌐

date:

weight:

MEAL #1

WHAT I ATE

CALORIES

TIME
OF DAY

HUNGER
BEFORE

HUNGER
AFTER

STARS: ☐ PROTEIN ☐ FIBER ☐ GOOD FATS ☐ FRUITS/VEGGIES

MEAL #2

WHAT I ATE

CALORIES

TIME
OF DAY

HUNGER
BEFORE

HUNGER
AFTER

STARS: ☐ PROTEIN ☐ FIBER ☐ GOOD FATS ☐ FRUITS/VEGGIES

MEAL #3

WHAT I ATE

CALORIES

TIME
OF DAY

HUNGER
BEFORE

HUNGER
AFTER

STARS: ☐ PROTEIN ☐ FIBER ☐ GOOD FATS ☐ FRUITS/VEGGIES

MEAL #4

WHAT I ATE

CALORIES	TIME OF DAY
HUNGER BEFORE	HUNGER AFTER

STARS: ☐ PROTEIN ☐ FIBER ☐ GOOD FATS ☐ FRUITS/VEGGIES

MEAL #5

WHAT I ATE

CALORIES	TIME OF DAY
HUNGER BEFORE	HUNGER AFTER

STARS: ☐ PROTEIN ☐ FIBER ☐ GOOD FATS ☐ FRUITS/VEGGIES

PHYSICAL ACTIVITY

Activity:
Duration:
Intensity:
Calories Burned:

Activity:
Duration:
Intensity:
Calories Burned:

OTHER NOTES

TOTAL CALORIES FOR THE DAY:

TOTAL STARS FOR THE DAY:

Protein

Fiber

Good Fats

Fruits/Veggies

400 CALORIE FIX TRACKER

date:

weight:

MEAL #1

WHAT I ATE

CALORIES

TIME
OF DAY

HUNGER
BEFORE

HUNGER
AFTER

STARS: ☐ PROTEIN ☐ FIBER ☐ GOOD FATS ☐ FRUITS/VEGGIES

MEAL #2

WHAT I ATE

CALORIES

TIME
OF DAY

HUNGER
BEFORE

HUNGER
AFTER

STARS: ☐ PROTEIN ☐ FIBER ☐ GOOD FATS ☐ FRUITS/VEGGIES

MEAL #3

WHAT I ATE

CALORIES

TIME
OF DAY

HUNGER
BEFORE

HUNGER
AFTER

STARS: ☐ PROTEIN ☐ FIBER ☐ GOOD FATS ☐ FRUITS/VEGGIES

MEAL #4

WHAT I ATE

CALORIES	TIME OF DAY
HUNGER BEFORE	HUNGER AFTER

STARS: ❑ PROTEIN ❑ FIBER ❑ GOOD FATS ❑ FRUITS/VEGGIES

MEAL #5

WHAT I ATE

CALORIES	TIME OF DAY
HUNGER BEFORE	HUNGER AFTER

STARS: ❑ PROTEIN ❑ FIBER ❑ GOOD FATS ❑ FRUITS/VEGGIES

PHYSICAL ACTIVITY

Activity:
Duration:
Intensity:
Calories Burned:

Activity:
Duration:
Intensity:
Calories Burned:

OTHER NOTES

TOTAL CALORIES FOR THE DAY:

TOTAL STARS FOR THE DAY:

Protein
❑ ❑ ❑ ❑
——————
Fiber
❑ ❑ ❑ ❑
——————
Good Fats
❑ ❑ ❑ ❑
——————
Fruits/Veggies
❑ ❑ ❑ ❑

date:

weight:

MEAL #1

WHAT I ATE

CALORIES

TIME OF DAY

HUNGER BEFORE

HUNGER AFTER

STARS: ☐ PROTEIN ☐ FIBER ☐ GOOD FATS ☐ FRUITS/VEGGIES

MEAL #2

WHAT I ATE

CALORIES

TIME OF DAY

HUNGER BEFORE

HUNGER AFTER

STARS: ☐ PROTEIN ☐ FIBER ☐ GOOD FATS ☐ FRUITS/VEGGIES

MEAL #3

WHAT I ATE

CALORIES

TIME OF DAY

HUNGER BEFORE

HUNGER AFTER

STARS: ☐ PROTEIN ☐ FIBER ☐ GOOD FATS ☐ FRUITS/VEGGIES

MEAL #4

WHAT I ATE

CALORIES	TIME OF DAY

HUNGER BEFORE	HUNGER AFTER

STARS: ❏ PROTEIN ❏ FIBER ❏ GOOD FATS ❏ FRUITS/VEGGIES

MEAL #5

WHAT I ATE

CALORIES	TIME OF DAY

HUNGER BEFORE	HUNGER AFTER

STARS: ❏ PROTEIN ❏ FIBER ❏ GOOD FATS ❏ FRUITS/VEGGIES

PHYSICAL ACTIVITY

Activity:
Duration:
Intensity:
Calories Burned:

Activity:
Duration:
Intensity:
Calories Burned:

OTHER NOTES

TOTAL CALORIES FOR THE DAY:

TOTAL STARS FOR THE DAY:

Protein
❏ ❏ ❏ ❏

Fiber
❏ ❏ ❏ ❏

Good Fats
❏ ❏ ❏ ❏

Fruits/Veggies
❏ ❏ ❏ ❏

date:

weight:

MEAL #1

WHAT I ATE

CALORIES

TIME OF DAY

HUNGER BEFORE

HUNGER AFTER

STARS: ☐ PROTEIN ☐ FIBER ☐ GOOD FATS ☐ FRUITS/VEGGIES

MEAL #2

WHAT I ATE

CALORIES

TIME OF DAY

HUNGER BEFORE

HUNGER AFTER

STARS: ☐ PROTEIN ☐ FIBER ☐ GOOD FATS ☐ FRUITS/VEGGIES

MEAL #3

WHAT I ATE

CALORIES

TIME OF DAY

HUNGER BEFORE

HUNGER AFTER

STARS: ☐ PROTEIN ☐ FIBER ☐ GOOD FATS ☐ FRUITS/VEGGIES

MEAL #4

WHAT I ATE

CALORIES	TIME OF DAY

HUNGER BEFORE	HUNGER AFTER

STARS: ❑ PROTEIN ❑ FIBER ❑ GOOD FATS ❑ FRUITS/VEGGIES

MEAL #5

WHAT I ATE

CALORIES	TIME OF DAY

HUNGER BEFORE	HUNGER AFTER

STARS: ❑ PROTEIN ❑ FIBER ❑ GOOD FATS ❑ FRUITS/VEGGIES

PHYSICAL ACTIVITY

Activity:
Duration:
Intensity:
Calories Burned:

Activity:
Duration:
Intensity:
Calories Burned:

OTHER NOTES

TOTAL CALORIES FOR THE DAY:

TOTAL STARS FOR THE DAY:

Protein
❑ ❑ ❑ ❑ ❑
_____

Fiber
❑ ❑ ❑ ❑ ❑
_____

Good Fats
❑ ❑ ❑ ❑ ❑
_____

Fruits/Veggies
❑ ❑ ❑ ❑ ❑

date:

weight:

MEAL #1

WHAT I ATE

CALORIES

TIME OF DAY

HUNGER BEFORE

HUNGER AFTER

STARS: ☐ PROTEIN ☐ FIBER ☐ GOOD FATS ☐ FRUITS/VEGGIES

MEAL #2

WHAT I ATE

CALORIES

TIME OF DAY

HUNGER BEFORE

HUNGER AFTER

STARS: ☐ PROTEIN ☐ FIBER ☐ GOOD FATS ☐ FRUITS/VEGGIES

MEAL #3

WHAT I ATE

CALORIES

TIME OF DAY

HUNGER BEFORE

HUNGER AFTER

STARS: ☐ PROTEIN ☐ FIBER ☐ GOOD FATS ☐ FRUITS/VEGGIES

MEAL #4

WHAT I ATE		
	CALORIES	TIME OF DAY
	HUNGER BEFORE	HUNGER AFTER

STARS: ☐ PROTEIN ☐ FIBER ☐ GOOD FATS ☐ FRUITS/VEGGIES

MEAL #5

WHAT I ATE		
	CALORIES	TIME OF DAY
	HUNGER BEFORE	HUNGER AFTER

STARS: ☐ PROTEIN ☐ FIBER ☐ GOOD FATS ☐ FRUITS/VEGGIES

PHYSICAL ACTIVITY

Activity:
Duration:
Intensity:
Calories Burned:

Activity:
Duration:
Intensity:
Calories Burned:

OTHER NOTES

TOTAL CALORIES FOR THE DAY:

TOTAL STARS FOR THE DAY.

Protein
☐ ☐ ☐ ☐ ☐

Fiber
☐ ☐ ☐ ☐ ☐

Good Fats
☐ ☐ ☐ ☐ ☐

Fruits/Veggies
☐ ☐ ☐ ☐ ☐

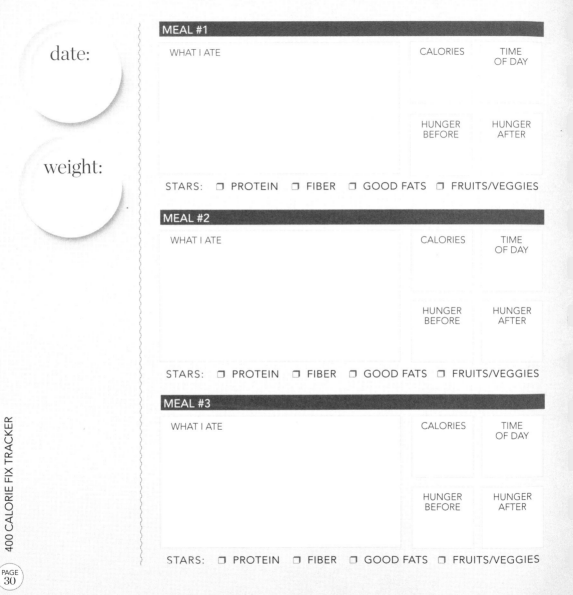

date:

weight:

MEAL #1

WHAT I ATE

CALORIES | TIME OF DAY

HUNGER BEFORE | HUNGER AFTER

STARS: ☐ PROTEIN ☐ FIBER ☐ GOOD FATS ☐ FRUITS/VEGGIES

MEAL #2

WHAT I ATE

CALORIES | TIME OF DAY

HUNGER BEFORE | HUNGER AFTER

STARS: ☐ PROTEIN ☐ FIBER ☐ GOOD FATS ☐ FRUITS/VEGGIES

MEAL #3

WHAT I ATE

CALORIES | TIME OF DAY

HUNGER BEFORE | HUNGER AFTER

STARS: ☐ PROTEIN ☐ FIBER ☐ GOOD FATS ☐ FRUITS/VEGGIES

MEAL #4

WHAT I ATE

CALORIES	TIME OF DAY
HUNGER BEFORE	HUNGER AFTER

STARS: ☐ PROTEIN ☐ FIBER ☐ GOOD FATS ☐ FRUITS/VEGGIES

MEAL #5

WHAT I ATE

CALORIES	TIME OF DAY
HUNGER BEFORE	HUNGER AFTER

STARS: ☐ PROTEIN ☐ FIBER ☐ GOOD FATS ☐ FRUITS/VEGGIES

PHYSICAL ACTIVITY

Activity:
Duration:
Intensity:
Calories Burned:

Activity:
Duration:
Intensity:
Calories Burned:

OTHER NOTES

TOTAL CALORIES FOR THE DAY:

TOTAL STARS FOR THE DAY:

Protein
☐ ☐ ☐ ☐ ☐
_____
Fiber
☐ ☐ ☐ ☐ ☐
_____
Good Fats
☐ ☐ ☐ ☐ ☐
_____
Fruits/Veggies
☐ ☐ ☐ ☐ ☐

date:

weight:

MEAL #1

WHAT I ATE

CALORIES

TIME
OF DAY

HUNGER
BEFORE

HUNGER
AFTER

STARS: ☐ PROTEIN ☐ FIBER ☐ GOOD FATS ☐ FRUITS/VEGGIES

MEAL #2

WHAT I ATE

CALORIES

TIME
OF DAY

HUNGER
BEFORE

HUNGER
AFTER

STARS: ☐ PROTEIN ☐ FIBER ☐ GOOD FATS ☐ FRUITS/VEGGIES

MEAL #3

WHAT I ATE

CALORIES

TIME
OF DAY

HUNGER
BEFORE

HUNGER
AFTER

STARS: ☐ PROTEIN ☐ FIBER ☐ GOOD FATS ☐ FRUITS/VEGGIES

MEAL #4

WHAT I ATE

CALORIES	TIME OF DAY

HUNGER BEFORE	HUNGER AFTER

STARS: ☐ PROTEIN ☐ FIBER ☐ GOOD FATS ☐ FRUITS/VEGGIES

MEAL #5

WHAT I ATE

CALORIES	TIME OF DAY

HUNGER BEFORE	HUNGER AFTER

STARS: ☐ PROTEIN ☐ FIBER ☐ GOOD FATS ☐ FRUITS/VEGGIES

PHYSICAL ACTIVITY

Activity:
Duration:
Intensity:
Calories Burned:

Activity:
Duration:
Intensity:
Calories Burned:

OTHER NOTES

TOTAL CALORIES FOR THE DAY:

TOTAL STARS FOR THE DAY:

Protein
☐ ☐ ☐ ☐

Fiber
☐ ☐ ☐ ☐

Good Fats
☐ ☐ ☐ ☐

Fruits/Veggies
☐ ☐ ☐ ☐

date:

weight:

MEAL #1

WHAT I ATE

CALORIES

TIME
OF DAY

HUNGER
BEFORE

HUNGER
AFTER

STARS: ☐ PROTEIN ☐ FIBER ☐ GOOD FATS ☐ FRUITS/VEGGIES

MEAL #2

WHAT I ATE

CALORIES

TIME
OF DAY

HUNGER
BEFORE

HUNGER
AFTER

STARS: ☐ PROTEIN ☐ FIBER ☐ GOOD FATS ☐ FRUITS/VEGGIES

MEAL #3

WHAT I ATE

CALORIES

TIME
OF DAY

HUNGER
BEFORE

HUNGER
AFTER

STARS: ☐ PROTEIN ☐ FIBER ☐ GOOD FATS ☐ FRUITS/VEGGIES

MEAL #4

WHAT I ATE

CALORIES	TIME OF DAY

HUNGER BEFORE	HUNGER AFTER

STARS: ☐ PROTEIN ☐ FIBER ☐ GOOD FATS ☐ FRUITS/VEGGIES

MEAL #5

WHAT I ATE

CALORIES	TIME OF DAY

HUNGER BEFORE	HUNGER AFTER

STARS: ☐ PROTEIN ☐ FIBER ☐ GOOD FATS ☐ FRUITS/VEGGIES

PHYSICAL ACTIVITY

Activity:
Duration:
Intensity:
Calories Burned:

Activity:
Duration:
Intensity:
Calories Burned:

OTHER NOTES

TOTAL CALORIES FOR THE DAY:

TOTAL STARS FOR THE DAY:

Protein
☐ ☐ ☐ ☐
_____

Fiber
☐ ☐ ☐ ☐
_____

Good Fats
☐ ☐ ☐ ☐
_____

Fruits/Veggies
☐ ☐ ☐ ☐

400 CALORIE FIX TRACKER

date:

weight:

MEAL #1

WHAT I ATE

CALORIES

TIME OF DAY

HUNGER BEFORE

HUNGER AFTER

STARS: ☐ PROTEIN ☐ FIBER ☐ GOOD FATS ☐ FRUITS/VEGGIES

MEAL #2

WHAT I ATE

CALORIES

TIME OF DAY

HUNGER BEFORE

HUNGER AFTER

STARS: ☐ PROTEIN ☐ FIBER ☐ GOOD FATS ☐ FRUITS/VEGGIES

MEAL #3

WHAT I ATE

CALORIES

TIME OF DAY

HUNGER BEFORE

HUNGER AFTER

STARS: ☐ PROTEIN ☐ FIBER ☐ GOOD FATS ☐ FRUITS/VEGGIES

MEAL #4

WHAT I ATE

CALORIES	TIME OF DAY

HUNGER BEFORE	HUNGER AFTER

STARS: ☐ PROTEIN ☐ FIBER ☐ GOOD FATS ☐ FRUITS/VEGGIES

MEAL #5

WHAT I ATE

CALORIES	TIME OF DAY

HUNGER BEFORE	HUNGER AFTER

STARS: ☐ PROTEIN ☐ FIBER ☐ GOOD FATS ☐ FRUITS/VEGGIES

PHYSICAL ACTIVITY

Activity:
Duration:
Intensity:
Calories Burned:

Activity:
Duration:
Intensity:
Calories Burned:

OTHER NOTES

TOTAL CALORIES FOR THE DAY:

TOTAL STARS FOR THE DAY:

Protein

☐ ☐ ☐ ☐ ☐
_____

Fiber

☐ ☐ ☐ ☐ ☐
_____

Good Fats

☐ ☐ ☐ ☐ ☐
_____

Fruits/Veggies

☐ ☐ ☐ ☐ ☐

date:

weight:

MEAL #1

WHAT I ATE

CALORIES

TIME
OF DAY

HUNGER
BEFORE

HUNGER
AFTER

STARS: ❑ PROTEIN   ❑ FIBER   ❑ GOOD FATS   ❑ FRUITS/VEGGIES

MEAL #2

WHAT I ATE

CALORIES

TIME
OF DAY

HUNGER
BEFORE

HUNGER
AFTER

STARS: ❑ PROTEIN   ❑ FIBER   ❑ GOOD FATS   ❑ FRUITS/VEGGIES

MEAL #3

WHAT I ATE

CALORIES

TIME
OF DAY

HUNGER
BEFORE

HUNGER
AFTER

STARS: ❑ PROTEIN   ❑ FIBER   ❑ GOOD FATS   ❑ FRUITS/VEGGIES

MEAL #4

WHAT I ATE

CALORIES	TIME OF DAY
HUNGER BEFORE	HUNGER AFTER

STARS: ☐ PROTEIN ☐ FIBER ☐ GOOD FATS ☐ FRUITS/VEGGIES

MEAL #5

WHAT I ATE

CALORIES	TIME OF DAY
HUNGER BEFORE	HUNGER AFTER

STARS: ☐ PROTEIN ☐ FIBER ☐ GOOD FATS ☐ FRUITS/VEGGIES

PHYSICAL ACTIVITY

Activity:
Duration:
Intensity:
Calories Burned:

Activity:
Duration:
Intensity:
Calories Burned:

OTHER NOTES

TOTAL CALORIES FOR THE DAY:

TOTAL STARS FOR THE DAY:

Protein

Fiber

Good Fats

Fruits/Veggies

date:

weight:

MEAL #1

WHAT I ATE

CALORIES

TIME
OF DAY

HUNGER
BEFORE

HUNGER
AFTER

STARS: ☐ PROTEIN ☐ FIBER ☐ GOOD FATS ☐ FRUITS/VEGGIES

MEAL #2

WHAT I ATE

CALORIES

TIME
OF DAY

HUNGER
BEFORE

HUNGER
AFTER

STARS: ☐ PROTEIN ☐ FIBER ☐ GOOD FATS ☐ FRUITS/VEGGIES

MEAL #3

WHAT I ATE

CALORIES

TIME
OF DAY

HUNGER
BEFORE

HUNGER
AFTER

STARS: ☐ PROTEIN ☐ FIBER ☐ GOOD FATS ☐ FRUITS/VEGGIES

MEAL #4

WHAT I ATE

CALORIES	TIME OF DAY

HUNGER BEFORE	HUNGER AFTER

STARS: ☐ PROTEIN ☐ FIBER ☐ GOOD FATS ☐ FRUITS/VEGGIES

MEAL #5

WHAT I ATE

CALORIES	TIME OF DAY

HUNGER BEFORE	HUNGER AFTER

STARS: ☐ PROTEIN ☐ FIBER ☐ GOOD FATS ☐ FRUITS/VEGGIES

PHYSICAL ACTIVITY

Activity:
Duration:
Intensity:
Calories Burned:

Activity:
Duration:
Intensity:
Calories Burned:

OTHER NOTES

TOTAL CALORIES FOR THE DAY:

TOTAL STARS FOR THE DAY:

Protein

Fiber

Good Fats

Fruits/Veggies

date:

weight:

MEAL #1

WHAT I ATE		CALORIES	TIME OF DAY
		HUNGER BEFORE	HUNGER AFTER

STARS: ☐ PROTEIN ☐ FIBER ☐ GOOD FATS ☐ FRUITS/VEGGIES

MEAL #2

WHAT I ATE		CALORIES	TIME OF DAY
		HUNGER BEFORE	HUNGER AFTER

STARS: ☐ PROTEIN ☐ FIBER ☐ GOOD FATS ☐ FRUITS/VEGGIES

MEAL #3

WHAT I ATE		CALORIES	TIME OF DAY
		HUNGER BEFORE	HUNGER AFTER

STARS: ☐ PROTEIN ☐ FIBER ☐ GOOD FATS ☐ FRUITS/VEGGIES

MEAL #4

WHAT I ATE

CALORIES

TIME OF DAY

HUNGER BEFORE

HUNGER AFTER

STARS: ☐ PROTEIN ☐ FIBER ☐ GOOD FATS ☐ FRUITS/VEGGIES

MEAL #5

WHAT I ATE

CALORIES

TIME OF DAY

HUNGER BEFORE

HUNGER AFTER

STARS: ☐ PROTEIN ☐ FIBER ☐ GOOD FATS ☐ FRUITS/VEGGIES

PHYSICAL ACTIVITY

Activity:
Duration:
Intensity:
Calories Burned:

Activity:
Duration:
Intensity:
Calories Burned:

OTHER NOTES

TOTAL CALORIES FOR THE DAY:

TOTAL STARS FOR THE DAY:

Protein
☐ ☐ ☐ ☐ ☐
___
Fiber
☐ ☐ ☐ ☐ ☐
___
Good Fats
☐ ☐ ☐ ☐ ☐
___
Fruits/Veggies
☐ ☐ ☐ ☐ ☐

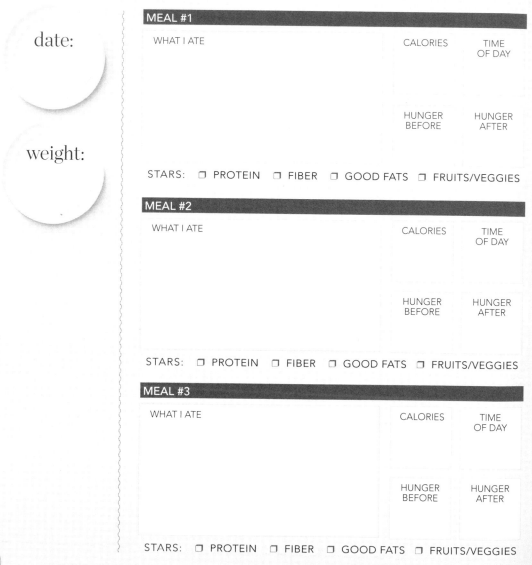

date:

weight:

MEAL #1

WHAT I ATE

CALORIES | TIME OF DAY

HUNGER BEFORE | HUNGER AFTER

STARS: ☐ PROTEIN ☐ FIBER ☐ GOOD FATS ☐ FRUITS/VEGGIES

MEAL #2

WHAT I ATE

CALORIES | TIME OF DAY

HUNGER BEFORE | HUNGER AFTER

STARS: ☐ PROTEIN ☐ FIBER ☐ GOOD FATS ☐ FRUITS/VEGGIES

MEAL #3

WHAT I ATE

CALORIES | TIME OF DAY

HUNGER BEFORE | HUNGER AFTER

STARS: ☐ PROTEIN ☐ FIBER ☐ GOOD FATS ☐ FRUITS/VEGGIES

400 CALORIE FIX TRACKER

MEAL #4

WHAT I ATE

CALORIES	TIME OF DAY

HUNGER BEFORE	HUNGER AFTER

STARS: ☐ PROTEIN ☐ FIBER ☐ GOOD FATS ☐ FRUITS/VEGGIES

MEAL #5

WHAT I ATE

CALORIES	TIME OF DAY

HUNGER BEFORE	HUNGER AFTER

STARS: ☐ PROTEIN ☐ FIBER ☐ GOOD FATS ☐ FRUITS/VEGGIES

PHYSICAL ACTIVITY

Activity:
Duration:
Intensity:
Calories Burned:

Activity:
Duration:
Intensity:
Calories Burned:

OTHER NOTES

TOTAL CALORIES FOR THE DAY:

TOTAL STARS FOR THE DAY:

Protein
☐ ☐ ☐ ☐

Fiber
☐ ☐ ☐ ☐

Good Fats
☐ ☐ ☐ ☐

Fruits/Veggies
☐ ☐ ☐ ☐

date:

weight:

MEAL #1

WHAT I ATE

CALORIES

TIME OF DAY

HUNGER BEFORE

HUNGER AFTER

STARS: ☐ PROTEIN ☐ FIBER ☐ GOOD FATS ☐ FRUITS/VEGGIES

MEAL #2

WHAT I ATE

CALORIES

TIME OF DAY

HUNGER BEFORE

HUNGER AFTER

STARS: ☐ PROTEIN ☐ FIBER ☐ GOOD FATS ☐ FRUITS/VEGGIES

MEAL #3

WHAT I ATE

CALORIES

TIME OF DAY

HUNGER BEFORE

HUNGER AFTER

STARS: ☐ PROTEIN ☐ FIBER ☐ GOOD FATS ☐ FRUITS/VEGGIES

MEAL #4

WHAT I ATE

CALORIES	TIME OF DAY

HUNGER BEFORE	HUNGER AFTER

STARS: ☐ PROTEIN ☐ FIBER ☐ GOOD FATS ☐ FRUITS/VEGGIES

MEAL #5

WHAT I ATE

CALORIES	TIME OF DAY

HUNGER BEFORE	HUNGER AFTER

STARS: ☐ PROTEIN ☐ FIBER ☐ GOOD FATS ☐ FRUITS/VEGGIES

PHYSICAL ACTIVITY

Activity:
Duration:
Intensity:
Calories Burned:

Activity:
Duration:
Intensity:
Calories Burned:

OTHER NOTES

TOTAL CALORIES FOR THE DAY:

TOTAL STARS FOR THE DAY:

Protein
☐ ☐ ☐ ☐
_____

Fiber
☐ ☐ ☐ ☐
_____

Good Fats
☐ ☐ ☐ ☐
_____

Fruits/Veggies
☐ ☐ ☐ ☐

date:

weight:

MEAL #1

WHAT I ATE

CALORIES | TIME OF DAY

HUNGER BEFORE | HUNGER AFTER

STARS: ☐ PROTEIN ☐ FIBER ☐ GOOD FATS ☐ FRUITS/VEGGIES

MEAL #2

WHAT I ATE

CALORIES | TIME OF DAY

HUNGER BEFORE | HUNGER AFTER

STARS: ☐ PROTEIN ☐ FIBER ☐ GOOD FATS ☐ FRUITS/VEGGIES

MEAL #3

WHAT I ATE

CALORIES | TIME OF DAY

HUNGER BEFORE | HUNGER AFTER

STARS: ☐ PROTEIN ☐ FIBER ☐ GOOD FATS ☐ FRUITS/VEGGIES

MEAL #4

WHAT I ATE

CALORIES	TIME OF DAY

HUNGER BEFORE	HUNGER AFTER

STARS: ☐ PROTEIN ☐ FIBER ☐ GOOD FATS ☐ FRUITS/VEGGIES

MEAL #5

WHAT I ATE

CALORIES	TIME OF DAY

HUNGER BEFORE	HUNGER AFTER

STARS: ☐ PROTEIN ☐ FIBER ☐ GOOD FATS ☐ FRUITS/VEGGIES

PHYSICAL ACTIVITY

Activity:
Duration:
Intensity:
Calories Burned:

Activity:
Duration:
Intensity:
Calories Burned:

OTHER NOTES

TOTAL CALORIES FOR THE DAY:

TOTAL STARS FOR THE DAY:

Protein
_____

Fiber
_____

Good Fats
_____

Fruits/Veggies

date:

weight:

MEAL #1

WHAT I ATE

CALORIES   TIME OF DAY

HUNGER BEFORE   HUNGER AFTER

STARS: ☐ PROTEIN ☐ FIBER ☐ GOOD FATS ☐ FRUITS/VEGGIES

MEAL #2

WHAT I ATE

CALORIES   TIME OF DAY

HUNGER BEFORE   HUNGER AFTER

STARS: ☐ PROTEIN ☐ FIBER ☐ GOOD FATS ☐ FRUITS/VEGGIES

MEAL #3

WHAT I ATE

CALORIES   TIME OF DAY

HUNGER BEFORE   HUNGER AFTER

STARS: ☐ PROTEIN ☐ FIBER ☐ GOOD FATS ☐ FRUITS/VEGGIES

MEAL #4

WHAT I ATE

CALORIES	TIME OF DAY

HUNGER BEFORE	HUNGER AFTER

STARS: ❏ PROTEIN ❏ FIBER ❏ GOOD FATS ❏ FRUITS/VEGGIES

MEAL #5

WHAT I ATE

CALORIES	TIME OF DAY

HUNGER BEFORE	HUNGER AFTER

STARS: ❏ PROTEIN ❏ FIBER ❏ GOOD FATS ❏ FRUITS/VEGGIES

PHYSICAL ACTIVITY

Activity:
Duration:
Intensity:
Calories Burned:

Activity:
Duration:
Intensity:
Calories Burned:

OTHER NOTES

TOTAL CALORIES FOR THE DAY:

TOTAL STARS FOR THE DAY:

Protein

Fiber

Good Fats

Fruits/Veggies

date:

weight:

MEAL #1

WHAT I ATE

CALORIES

TIME OF DAY

HUNGER BEFORE

HUNGER AFTER

STARS: ☐ PROTEIN ☐ FIBER ☐ GOOD FATS ☐ FRUITS/VEGGIES

MEAL #2

WHAT I ATE

CALORIES

TIME OF DAY

HUNGER BEFORE

HUNGER AFTER

STARS: ☐ PROTEIN ☐ FIBER ☐ GOOD FATS ☐ FRUITS/VEGGIES

MEAL #3

WHAT I ATE

CALORIES

TIME OF DAY

HUNGER BEFORE

HUNGER AFTER

STARS: ☐ PROTEIN ☐ FIBER ☐ GOOD FATS ☐ FRUITS/VEGGIES

MEAL #4

WHAT I ATE

CALORIES	TIME OF DAY

HUNGER BEFORE	HUNGER AFTER

STARS: ☐ PROTEIN ☐ FIBER ☐ GOOD FATS ☐ FRUITS/VEGGIES

MEAL #5

WHAT I ATE

CALORIES	TIME OF DAY

HUNGER BEFORE	HUNGER AFTER

STARS: ☐ PROTEIN ☐ FIBER ☐ GOOD FATS ☐ FRUITS/VEGGIES

PHYSICAL ACTIVITY

Activity:
Duration:
Intensity:
Calories Burned:

Activity:
Duration:
Intensity:
Calories Burned:

OTHER NOTES

TOTAL CALORIES FOR THE DAY:

TOTAL STARS FOR THE DAY:

Protein

Fiber

Good Fats

Fruits/Veggies

date:

weight:

MEAL #1

WHAT I ATE

CALORIES   TIME
OF DAY

HUNGER   HUNGER
BEFORE   AFTER

STARS: ☐ PROTEIN ☐ FIBER ☐ GOOD FATS ☐ FRUITS/VEGGIES

MEAL #2

WHAT I ATE

CALORIES   TIME
OF DAY

HUNGER   HUNGER
BEFORE   AFTER

STARS: ☐ PROTEIN ☐ FIBER ☐ GOOD FATS ☐ FRUITS/VEGGIES

MEAL #3

WHAT I ATE

CALORIES   TIME
OF DAY

HUNGER   HUNGER
BEFORE   AFTER

STARS: ☐ PROTEIN ☐ FIBER ☐ GOOD FATS ☐ FRUITS/VEGGIES

MEAL #4

WHAT I ATE

CALORIES	TIME OF DAY
HUNGER BEFORE	HUNGER AFTER

STARS: ☐ PROTEIN ☐ FIBER ☐ GOOD FATS ☐ FRUITS/VEGGIES

MEAL #5

WHAT I ATE

CALORIES	TIME OF DAY
HUNGER BEFORE	HUNGER AFTER

STARS: ☐ PROTEIN ☐ FIBER ☐ GOOD FATS ☐ FRUITS/VEGGIES

PHYSICAL ACTIVITY

Activity:
Duration:
Intensity:
Calories Burned:

Activity:
Duration:
Intensity:
Calories Burned:

OTHER NOTES

TOTAL CALORIES FOR THE DAY:

TOTAL STARS FOR THE DAY:

Protein

Fiber

Good Fats

Fruits/Veggies

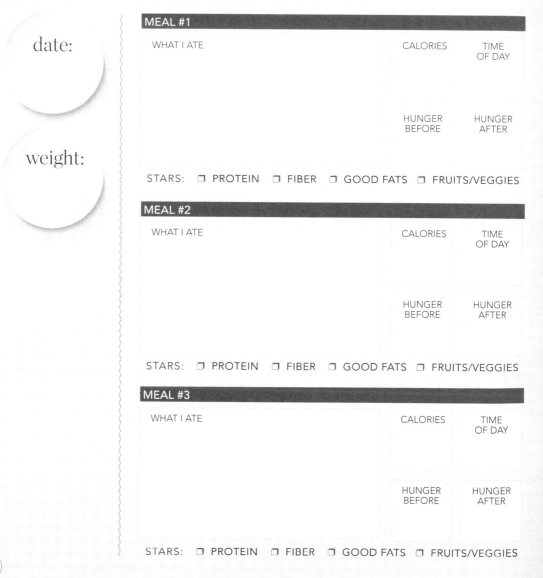

date:

weight:

MEAL #1

WHAT I ATE

CALORIES

TIME OF DAY

HUNGER BEFORE

HUNGER AFTER

STARS: ☐ PROTEIN ☐ FIBER ☐ GOOD FATS ☐ FRUITS/VEGGIES

MEAL #2

WHAT I ATE

CALORIES

TIME OF DAY

HUNGER BEFORE

HUNGER AFTER

STARS: ☐ PROTEIN ☐ FIBER ☐ GOOD FATS ☐ FRUITS/VEGGIES

MEAL #3

WHAT I ATE

CALORIES

TIME OF DAY

HUNGER BEFORE

HUNGER AFTER

STARS: ☐ PROTEIN ☐ FIBER ☐ GOOD FATS ☐ FRUITS/VEGGIES

MEAL #4

WHAT I ATE

CALORIES	TIME OF DAY
HUNGER BEFORE	HUNGER AFTER

STARS: ☐ PROTEIN ☐ FIBER ☐ GOOD FATS ☐ FRUITS/VEGGIES

MEAL #5

WHAT I ATE

CALORIES	TIME OF DAY
HUNGER BEFORE	HUNGER AFTER

STARS: ☐ PROTEIN ☐ FIBER ☐ GOOD FATS ☐ FRUITS/VEGGIES

PHYSICAL ACTIVITY

Activity:
Duration:
Intensity:
Calories Burned:

Activity:
Duration:
Intensity:
Calories Burned:

OTHER NOTES

TOTAL CALORIES FOR THE DAY:

TOTAL STARS FOR THE DAY:

Protein
☐ ☐ ☐ ☐
_____
Fiber
☐ ☐ ☐ ☐
_____
Good Fats
☐ ☐ ☐ ☐
_____
Fruits/Veggies
☐ ☐ ☐ ☐

400 CALORIE FIX TRACKER

date:

weight:

MEAL #1

WHAT I ATE   CALORIES TIME
OF DAY

HUNGER HUNGER
BEFORE AFTER

STARS: ❐ PROTEIN ❐ FIBER ❐ GOOD FATS ❐ FRUITS/VEGGIES

MEAL #2

WHAT I ATE   CALORIES TIME
OF DAY

HUNGER HUNGER
BEFORE AFTER

STARS: ❐ PROTEIN ❐ FIBER ❐ GOOD FATS ❐ FRUITS/VEGGIES

MEAL #3

WHAT I ATE   CALORIES TIME
OF DAY

HUNGER HUNGER
BEFORE AFTER

STARS: ❐ PROTEIN ❐ FIBER ❐ GOOD FATS ❐ FRUITS/VEGGIES

MEAL #4

WHAT I ATE

CALORIES

TIME OF DAY

HUNGER BEFORE

HUNGER AFTER

STARS: ☐ PROTEIN ☐ FIBER ☐ GOOD FATS ☐ FRUITS/VEGGIES

MEAL #5

WHAT I ATE

CALORIES

TIME OF DAY

HUNGER BEFORE

HUNGER AFTER

STARS: ☐ PROTEIN ☐ FIBER ☐ GOOD FATS ☐ FRUITS/VEGGIES

PHYSICAL ACTIVITY

Activity:
Duration:
Intensity:
Calories Burned:

Activity:
Duration:
Intensity:
Calories Burned:

OTHER NOTES

TOTAL CALORIES FOR THE DAY:

TOTAL STARS FOR THE DAY:

Protein

☐ ☐ ☐ ☐
_____

Fiber

☐ ☐ ☐ ☐
_____

Good Fats

☐ ☐ ☐ ☐
_____

Fruits/Veggies

☐ ☐ ☐ ☐

date:

weight:

MEAL #1

WHAT I ATE

CALORIES

TIME
OF DAY

HUNGER
BEFORE

HUNGER
AFTER

STARS: ☐ PROTEIN ☐ FIBER ☐ GOOD FATS ☐ FRUITS/VEGGIES

MEAL #2

WHAT I ATE

CALORIES

TIME
OF DAY

HUNGER
BEFORE

HUNGER
AFTER

STARS: ☐ PROTEIN ☐ FIBER ☐ GOOD FATS ☐ FRUITS/VEGGIES

MEAL #3

WHAT I ATE

CALORIES

TIME
OF DAY

HUNGER
BEFORE

HUNGER
AFTER

STARS: ☐ PROTEIN ☐ FIBER ☐ GOOD FATS ☐ FRUITS/VEGGIES

MEAL #4

WHAT I ATE

CALORIES	TIME OF DAY

HUNGER BEFORE	HUNGER AFTER

STARS: ☐ PROTEIN ☐ FIBER ☐ GOOD FATS ☐ FRUITS/VEGGIES

MEAL #5

WHAT I ATE

CALORIES	TIME OF DAY

HUNGER BEFORE	HUNGER AFTER

STARS: ☐ PROTEIN ☐ FIBER ☐ GOOD FATS ☐ FRUITS/VEGGIES

PHYSICAL ACTIVITY

Activity:
Duration:
Intensity:
Calories Burned:

Activity:
Duration:
Intensity:
Calories Burned:

OTHER NOTES

TOTAL CALORIES FOR THE DAY:

TOTAL STARS FOR THE DAY:

Protein
☐ ☐ ☐ ☐

Fiber
☐ ☐ ☐ ☐

Good Fats
☐ ☐ ☐ ☐

Fruits/Veggies
☐ ☐ ☐ ☐

date:

weight:

MEAL #1

WHAT I ATE

CALORIES | TIME OF DAY

HUNGER BEFORE | HUNGER AFTER

STARS: ☐ PROTEIN ☐ FIBER ☐ GOOD FATS ☐ FRUITS/VEGGIES

MEAL #2

WHAT I ATE

CALORIES | TIME OF DAY

HUNGER BEFORE | HUNGER AFTER

STARS: ☐ PROTEIN ☐ FIBER ☐ GOOD FATS ☐ FRUITS/VEGGIES

MEAL #3

WHAT I ATE

CALORIES | TIME OF DAY

HUNGER BEFORE | HUNGER AFTER

STARS: ☐ PROTEIN ☐ FIBER ☐ GOOD FATS ☐ FRUITS/VEGGIES

MEAL #4

WHAT I ATE

CALORIES	TIME OF DAY

HUNGER BEFORE	HUNGER AFTER

STARS: ☐ PROTEIN   ☐ FIBER   ☐ GOOD FATS   ☐ FRUITS/VEGGIES

MEAL #5

WHAT I ATE

CALORIES	TIME OF DAY

HUNGER BEFORE	HUNGER AFTER

STARS: ☐ PROTEIN   ☐ FIBER   ☐ GOOD FATS   ☐ FRUITS/VEGGIES

PHYSICAL ACTIVITY

Activity:
Duration:
Intensity:
Calories Burned:

Activity:
Duration:
Intensity:
Calories Burned:

OTHER NOTES

TOTAL CALORIES FOR THE DAY:

TOTAL STARS FOR THE DAY:

Protein
☐ ☐ ☐ ☐ ☐
_____
Fiber
☐ ☐ ☐ ☐ ☐
_____
Good Fats
☐ ☐ ☐ ☐ ☐
_____
Fruits/Veggies
☐ ☐ ☐ ☐ ☐

date:

weight:

MEAL #1

WHAT I ATE

CALORIES

TIME
OF DAY

HUNGER
BEFORE

HUNGER
AFTER

STARS: ☐ PROTEIN ☐ FIBER ☐ GOOD FATS ☐ FRUITS/VEGGIES

MEAL #2

WHAT I ATE

CALORIES

TIME
OF DAY

HUNGER
BEFORE

HUNGER
AFTER

STARS: ☐ PROTEIN ☐ FIBER ☐ GOOD FATS ☐ FRUITS/VEGGIES

MEAL #3

WHAT I ATE

CALORIES

TIME
OF DAY

HUNGER
BEFORE

HUNGER
AFTER

STARS: ☐ PROTEIN ☐ FIBER ☐ GOOD FATS ☐ FRUITS/VEGGIES

MEAL #4

WHAT I ATE	CALORIES	TIME OF DAY
	HUNGER BEFORE	HUNGER AFTER

STARS: ☐ PROTEIN ☐ FIBER ☐ GOOD FATS ☐ FRUITS/VEGGIES

MEAL #5

WHAT I ATE	CALORIES	TIME OF DAY
	HUNGER BEFORE	HUNGER AFTER

STARS: ☐ PROTEIN ☐ FIBER ☐ GOOD FATS ☐ FRUITS/VEGGIES

PHYSICAL ACTIVITY

Activity:
Duration:
Intensity:
Calories Burned:

Activity:
Duration:
Intensity:
Calories Burned:

OTHER NOTES

TOTAL
CALORIES
FOR THE DAY:

TOTAL STARS
FOR THE DAY:

Protein
☐ ☐ ☐ ☐ ☐

Fiber
☐ ☐ ☐ ☐ ☐

Good Fats
☐ ☐ ☐ ☐ ☐

Fruits/Veggies
☐ ☐ ☐ ☐ ☐

date:

weight:

MEAL #1

WHAT I ATE

CALORIES	TIME OF DAY
HUNGER BEFORE	HUNGER AFTER

STARS: ☐ PROTEIN ☐ FIBER ☐ GOOD FATS ☐ FRUITS/VEGGIES

MEAL #2

WHAT I ATE

CALORIES	TIME OF DAY
HUNGER BEFORE	HUNGER AFTER

STARS: ☐ PROTEIN ☐ FIBER ☐ GOOD FATS ☐ FRUITS/VEGGIES

MEAL #3

WHAT I ATE

CALORIES	TIME OF DAY
HUNGER BEFORE	HUNGER AFTER

STARS: ☐ PROTEIN ☐ FIBER ☐ GOOD FATS ☐ FRUITS/VEGGIES

MEAL #4

WHAT I ATE

CALORIES	TIME OF DAY

HUNGER BEFORE	HUNGER AFTER

STARS: ☐ PROTEIN ☐ FIBER ☐ GOOD FATS ☐ FRUITS/VEGGIES

MEAL #5

WHAT I ATE

CALORIES	TIME OF DAY

HUNGER BEFORE	HUNGER AFTER

STARS: ☐ PROTEIN ☐ FIBER ☐ GOOD FATS ☐ FRUITS/VEGGIES

PHYSICAL ACTIVITY

Activity:
Duration:
Intensity:
Calories Burned:

Activity:
Duration:
Intensity:
Calories Burned:

OTHER NOTES

TOTAL CALORIES FOR THE DAY:

TOTAL STARS FOR THE DAY:

Protein

Fiber

Good Fats

Fruits/Veggies

date:

weight:

MEAL #1

WHAT I ATE

CALORIES

TIME
OF DAY

HUNGER
BEFORE

HUNGER
AFTER

STARS: ☐ PROTEIN ☐ FIBER ☐ GOOD FATS ☐ FRUITS/VEGGIES

MEAL #2

WHAT I ATE

CALORIES

TIME
OF DAY

HUNGER
BEFORE

HUNGER
AFTER

STARS: ☐ PROTEIN ☐ FIBER ☐ GOOD FATS ☐ FRUITS/VEGGIES

MEAL #3

WHAT I ATE

CALORIES

TIME
OF DAY

HUNGER
BEFORE

HUNGER
AFTER

STARS: ☐ PROTEIN ☐ FIBER ☐ GOOD FATS ☐ FRUITS/VEGGIES

MEAL #4

WHAT I ATE

CALORIES	TIME OF DAY
HUNGER BEFORE	HUNGER AFTER

STARS: ☐ PROTEIN ☐ FIBER ☐ GOOD FATS ☐ FRUITS/VEGGIES

MEAL #5

WHAT I ATE

CALORIES	TIME OF DAY
HUNGER BEFORE	HUNGER AFTER

STARS: ☐ PROTEIN ☐ FIBER ☐ GOOD FATS ☐ FRUITS/VEGGIES

PHYSICAL ACTIVITY

Activity:
Duration:
Intensity:
Calories Burned:

Activity:
Duration:
Intensity:
Calories Burned:

OTHER NOTES

TOTAL CALORIES FOR THE DAY:

TOTAL STARS FOR THE DAY:

Protein
☐ ☐ ☐ ☐ ☐
_____
Fiber
☐ ☐ ☐ ☐ ☐
_____
Good Fats
☐ ☐ ☐ ☐ ☐
_____
Fruits/Veggies
☐ ☐ ☐ ☐ ☐

date:

weight:

MEAL #1

WHAT I ATE

CALORIES	TIME OF DAY
HUNGER BEFORE	HUNGER AFTER

STARS: ☐ PROTEIN ☐ FIBER ☐ GOOD FATS ☐ FRUITS/VEGGIES

MEAL #2

WHAT I ATE

CALORIES	TIME OF DAY
HUNGER BEFORE	HUNGER AFTER

STARS: ☐ PROTEIN ☐ FIBER ☐ GOOD FATS ☐ FRUITS/VEGGIES

MEAL #3

WHAT I ATE

CALORIES	TIME OF DAY
HUNGER BEFORE	HUNGER AFTER

STARS: ☐ PROTEIN ☐ FIBER ☐ GOOD FATS ☐ FRUITS/VEGGIES

MEAL #4

WHAT I ATE

CALORIES

TIME OF DAY

HUNGER BEFORE

HUNGER AFTER

STARS: ☐ PROTEIN ☐ FIBER ☐ GOOD FATS ☐ FRUITS/VEGGIES

MEAL #5

WHAT I ATE

CALORIES

TIME OF DAY

HUNGER BEFORE

HUNGER AFTER

STARS: ☐ PROTEIN ☐ FIBER ☐ GOOD FATS ☐ FRUITS/VEGGIES

PHYSICAL ACTIVITY

Activity:
Duration:
Intensity:
Calories Burned:

Activity:
Duration:
Intensity:
Calories Burned:

OTHER NOTES

TOTAL CALORIES FOR THE DAY:

TOTAL STARS FOR THE DAY:

Protein

⊓ ⊓ ⊓ ⊓ ⊓
_____

Fiber

⊓ ⊓ ⊓ ⊓ ⊓
_____

Good Fats

⊓ ⊓ ⊓ ⊓ ⊓

Fruits/Veggies

⊓ ⊓ ⊓ ⊓ ⊓

date:

weight:

MEAL #1

WHAT I ATE

CALORIES   TIME
OF DAY

HUNGER   HUNGER
BEFORE   AFTER

STARS: ☐ PROTEIN   ☐ FIBER   ☐ GOOD FATS   ☐ FRUITS/VEGGIES

MEAL #2

WHAT I ATE

CALORIES   TIME
OF DAY

HUNGER   HUNGER
BEFORE   AFTER

STARS: ☐ PROTEIN   ☐ FIBER   ☐ GOOD FATS   ☐ FRUITS/VEGGIES

MEAL #3

WHAT I ATE

CALORIES   TIME
OF DAY

HUNGER   HUNGER
BEFORE   AFTER

STARS: ☐ PROTEIN   ☐ FIBER   ☐ GOOD FATS   ☐ FRUITS/VEGGIES

MEAL #4

WHAT I ATE

CALORIES

TIME OF DAY

HUNGER BEFORE

HUNGER AFTER

STARS: ☐ PROTEIN ☐ FIBER ☐ GOOD FATS ☐ FRUITS/VEGGIES

MEAL #5

WHAT I ATE

CALORIES

TIME OF DAY

HUNGER BEFORE

HUNGER AFTER

STARS: ☐ PROTEIN ☐ FIBER ☐ GOOD FATS ☐ FRUITS/VEGGIES

PHYSICAL ACTIVITY

Activity:
Duration:
Intensity:
Calories Burned:

Activity:
Duration:
Intensity:
Calories Burned:

OTHER NOTES

TOTAL CALORIES FOR THE DAY:

TOTAL STARS FOR THE DAY:

Protein
☐ ☐ ☐ ☐
___
Fiber
☐ ☐ ☐ ☐
___
Good Fats
☐ ☐ ☐ ☐
___
Fruits/Veggies
☐ ☐ ☐ ☐

400 CALORIE FIX TRACKER

date:

weight:

MEAL #1

WHAT I ATE

CALORIES

TIME
OF DAY

HUNGER
BEFORE

HUNGER
AFTER

STARS: ☐ PROTEIN ☐ FIBER ☐ GOOD FATS ☐ FRUITS/VEGGIES

MEAL #2

WHAT I ATE

CALORIES

TIME
OF DAY

HUNGER
BEFORE

HUNGER
AFTER

STARS: ☐ PROTEIN ☐ FIBER ☐ GOOD FATS ☐ FRUITS/VEGGIES

MEAL #3

WHAT I ATE

CALORIES

TIME
OF DAY

HUNGER
BEFORE

HUNGER
AFTER

STARS: ☐ PROTEIN ☐ FIBER ☐ GOOD FATS ☐ FRUITS/VEGGIES

MEAL #4

WHAT I ATE

CALORIES	TIME OF DAY

HUNGER BEFORE	HUNGER AFTER

STARS: ☐ PROTEIN ☐ FIBER ☐ GOOD FATS ☐ FRUITS/VEGGIES

MEAL #5

WHAT I ATE

CALORIES	TIME OF DAY

HUNGER BEFORE	HUNGER AFTER

STARS: ☐ PROTEIN ☐ FIBER ☐ GOOD FATS ☐ FRUITS/VEGGIES

PHYSICAL ACTIVITY

Activity:
Duration:
Intensity:
Calories Burned:

Activity:
Duration:
Intensity:
Calories Burned:

OTHER NOTES

TOTAL CALORIES FOR THE DAY:

TOTAL STARS FOR THE DAY:

Protein
☐☐☐☐☐

Fiber
☐☐☐☐☐

Good Fats
☐☐☐☐☐

Fruits/Veggies
☐☐☐☐☐

date:

weight:

MEAL #1

WHAT I ATE

CALORIES | TIME OF DAY

HUNGER BEFORE | HUNGER AFTER

STARS: ☐ PROTEIN ☐ FIBER ☐ GOOD FATS ☐ FRUITS/VEGGIES

MEAL #2

WHAT I ATE

CALORIES | TIME OF DAY

HUNGER BEFORE | HUNGER AFTER

STARS: ☐ PROTEIN ☐ FIBER ☐ GOOD FATS ☐ FRUITS/VEGGIES

MEAL #3

WHAT I ATE

CALORIES | TIME OF DAY

HUNGER BEFORE | HUNGER AFTER

STARS: ☐ PROTEIN ☐ FIBER ☐ GOOD FATS ☐ FRUITS/VEGGIES

MEAL #4

WHAT I ATE

CALORIES	TIME OF DAY

HUNGER BEFORE	HUNGER AFTER

STARS: ☐ PROTEIN ☐ FIBER ☐ GOOD FATS ☐ FRUITS/VEGGIES

MEAL #5

WHAT I ATE

CALORIES	TIME OF DAY

HUNGER BEFORE	HUNGER AFTER

STARS: ☐ PROTEIN ☐ FIBER ☐ GOOD FATS ☐ FRUITS/VEGGIES

PHYSICAL ACTIVITY

Activity:
Duration:
Intensity:
Calories Burned:

Activity:
Duration:
Intensity:
Calories Burned:

OTHER NOTES

TOTAL CALORIES FOR THE DAY:

TOTAL STARS FOR THE DAY:

Protein
☐ ☐ ☐ ☐ ☐

Fiber
☐ ☐ ☐ ☐ ☐

Good Fats
☐ ☐ ☐ ☐ ☐

Fruits/Veggies
☐ ☐ ☐ ☐

date:

weight:

MEAL #1

WHAT I ATE

CALORIES | TIME OF DAY

HUNGER BEFORE | HUNGER AFTER

STARS: ☐ PROTEIN ☐ FIBER ☐ GOOD FATS ☐ FRUITS/VEGGIES

MEAL #2

WHAT I ATE

CALORIES | TIME OF DAY

HUNGER BEFORE | HUNGER AFTER

STARS: ☐ PROTEIN ☐ FIBER ☐ GOOD FATS ☐ FRUITS/VEGGIES

MEAL #3

WHAT I ATE

CALORIES | TIME OF DAY

HUNGER BEFORE | HUNGER AFTER

STARS: ☐ PROTEIN ☐ FIBER ☐ GOOD FATS ☐ FRUITS/VEGGIES

MEAL #4

WHAT I ATE

CALORIES	TIME OF DAY
HUNGER BEFORE	HUNGER AFTER

STARS: ☐ PROTEIN ☐ FIBER ☐ GOOD FATS ☐ FRUITS/VEGGIES

MEAL #5

WHAT I ATE

CALORIES	TIME OF DAY
HUNGER BEFORE	HUNGER AFTER

STARS: ☐ PROTEIN ☐ FIBER ☐ GOOD FATS ☐ FRUITS/VEGGIES

PHYSICAL ACTIVITY

Activity:
Duration:
Intensity:
Calories Burned:

Activity:
Duration:
Intensity:
Calories Burned:

OTHER NOTES

TOTAL CALORIES FOR THE DAY:

TOTAL STARS FOR THE DAY:

Protein
_____

Fiber
_____

Good Fats
_____

Fruits/Veggies

date:

weight:

MEAL #1

WHAT I ATE

CALORIES

TIME OF DAY

HUNGER BEFORE

HUNGER AFTER

STARS: ☐ PROTEIN ☐ FIBER ☐ GOOD FATS ☐ FRUITS/VEGGIES

MEAL #2

WHAT I ATE

CALORIES

TIME OF DAY

HUNGER BEFORE

HUNGER AFTER

STARS: ☐ PROTEIN ☐ FIBER ☐ GOOD FATS ☐ FRUITS/VEGGIES

MEAL #3

WHAT I ATE

CALORIES

TIME OF DAY

HUNGER BEFORE

HUNGER AFTER

STARS: ☐ PROTEIN ☐ FIBER ☐ GOOD FATS ☐ FRUITS/VEGGIES

MEAL #4

WHAT I ATE

CALORIES	TIME OF DAY
HUNGER BEFORE	HUNGER AFTER

STARS: ☐ PROTEIN ☐ FIBER ☐ GOOD FATS ☐ FRUITS/VEGGIES

MEAL #5

WHAT I ATE

CALORIES	TIME OF DAY
HUNGER BEFORE	HUNGER AFTER

STARS: ☐ PROTEIN ☐ FIBER ☐ GOOD FATS ☐ FRUITS/VEGGIES

PHYSICAL ACTIVITY

Activity:
Duration:
Intensity:
Calories Burned:

Activity:
Duration:
Intensity:
Calories Burned:

OTHER NOTES

TOTAL CALORIES FOR THE DAY:

TOTAL STARS FOR THE DAY:

Protein
☐ ☐ ☐ ☐ _____

Fiber
☐ ☐ ☐ ☐ _____

Good Fats
☐ ☐ ☐ ☐ _____

Fruits/Veggies
☐ ☐ ☐ ☐

date:

weight:

MEAL #1

WHAT I ATE

CALORIES | TIME OF DAY

HUNGER BEFORE | HUNGER AFTER

STARS: ☐ PROTEIN ☐ FIBER ☐ GOOD FATS ☐ FRUITS/VEGGIES

MEAL #2

WHAT I ATE

CALORIES | TIME OF DAY

HUNGER BEFORE | HUNGER AFTER

STARS: ☐ PROTEIN ☐ FIBER ☐ GOOD FATS ☐ FRUITS/VEGGIES

MEAL #3

WHAT I ATE

CALORIES | TIME OF DAY

HUNGER BEFORE | HUNGER AFTER

STARS: ☐ PROTEIN ☐ FIBER ☐ GOOD FATS ☐ FRUITS/VEGGIES

MEAL #4

WHAT I ATE

CALORIES

TIME OF DAY

HUNGER BEFORE

HUNGER AFTER

STARS: ☐ PROTEIN ☐ FIBER ☐ GOOD FATS ☐ FRUITS/VEGGIES

MEAL #5

WHAT I ATE

CALORIES

TIME OF DAY

HUNGER BEFORE

HUNGER AFTER

STARS: ☐ PROTEIN ☐ FIBER ☐ GOOD FATS ☐ FRUITS/VEGGIES

PHYSICAL ACTIVITY

Activity:
Duration:
Intensity:
Calories Burned:

Activity:
Duration:
Intensity:
Calories Burned:

OTHER NOTES

TOTAL CALORIES FOR THE DAY:

TOTAL STARS FOR THE DAY:

Protein

☐ ☐ ☐ ☐

Fiber

☐ ☐ ☐ ☐

Good Fats

☐ ☐ ☐ ☐

Fruits/Veggies

☐ ☐ ☐ ☐

date:

weight:

MEAL #1

WHAT I ATE

CALORIES

TIME
OF DAY

HUNGER
BEFORE

HUNGER
AFTER

STARS: ❏ PROTEIN ❏ FIBER ❏ GOOD FATS ❏ FRUITS/VEGGIES

MEAL #2

WHAT I ATE

CALORIES

TIME
OF DAY

HUNGER
BEFORE

HUNGER
AFTER

STARS: ❏ PROTEIN ❏ FIBER ❏ GOOD FATS ❏ FRUITS/VEGGIES

MEAL #3

WHAT I ATE

CALORIES

TIME
OF DAY

HUNGER
BEFORE

HUNGER
AFTER

STARS: ❏ PROTEIN ❏ FIBER ❏ GOOD FATS ❏ FRUITS/VEGGIES

MEAL #4

WHAT I ATE

CALORIES	TIME OF DAY

HUNGER BEFORE	HUNGER AFTER

STARS: ☐ PROTEIN   ☐ FIBER   ☐ GOOD FATS   ☐ FRUITS/VEGGIES

MEAL #5

WHAT I ATE

CALORIES	TIME OF DAY

HUNGER BEFORE	HUNGER AFTER

STARS: ☐ PROTEIN   ☐ FIBER   ☐ GOOD FATS   ☐ FRUITS/VEGGIES

PHYSICAL ACTIVITY

Activity:
Duration:
Intensity:
Calories Burned:

Activity:
Duration:
Intensity:
Calories Burned:

OTHER NOTES

TOTAL CALORIES FOR THE DAY:

TOTAL STARS FOR THE DAY:

Protein
⊓ ⊓ ⊓ ⊓ ⊓
_____

Fiber
⊓ ⊓ ⊓ ⊓ ⊓
_____

Good Fats
⊓ ⊓ ⊓ ⊓ ⊓
_____

Fruits/Veggies
⊓ ⊓ ⊓ ⊓ ⊓

date:

weight:

MEAL #1

WHAT I ATE

CALORIES

TIME OF DAY

HUNGER BEFORE

HUNGER AFTER

STARS: ☐ PROTEIN ☐ FIBER ☐ GOOD FATS ☐ FRUITS/VEGGIES

MEAL #2

WHAT I ATE

CALORIES

TIME OF DAY

HUNGER BEFORE

HUNGER AFTER

STARS: ☐ PROTEIN ☐ FIBER ☐ GOOD FATS ☐ FRUITS/VEGGIES

MEAL #3

WHAT I ATE

CALORIES

TIME OF DAY

HUNGER BEFORE

HUNGER AFTER

STARS: ☐ PROTEIN ☐ FIBER ☐ GOOD FATS ☐ FRUITS/VEGGIES

MEAL #4

WHAT I ATE

CALORIES	TIME OF DAY

HUNGER BEFORE	HUNGER AFTER

STARS: ☐ PROTEIN ☐ FIBER ☐ GOOD FATS ☐ FRUITS/VEGGIES

MEAL #5

WHAT I ATE

CALORIES	TIME OF DAY

HUNGER BEFORE	HUNGER AFTER

STARS: ☐ PROTEIN ☐ FIBER ☐ GOOD FATS ☐ FRUITS/VEGGIES

PHYSICAL ACTIVITY

Activity:
Duration:
Intensity:
Calories Burned:

Activity:
Duration:
Intensity:
Calories Burned:

OTHER NOTES

TOTAL CALORIES FOR THE DAY:

TOTAL STARS FOR THE DAY:

Protein

Fiber

Good Fats

Fruits/Veggies

date:

weight:

MEAL #1

WHAT I ATE

CALORIES   TIME OF DAY

HUNGER BEFORE   HUNGER AFTER

STARS: ☐ PROTEIN ☐ FIBER ☐ GOOD FATS ☐ FRUITS/VEGGIES

MEAL #2

WHAT I ATE

CALORIES   TIME OF DAY

HUNGER BEFORE   HUNGER AFTER

STARS: ☐ PROTEIN ☐ FIBER ☐ GOOD FATS ☐ FRUITS/VEGGIES

MEAL #3

WHAT I ATE

CALORIES   TIME OF DAY

HUNGER BEFORE   HUNGER AFTER

STARS: ☐ PROTEIN ☐ FIBER ☐ GOOD FATS ☐ FRUITS/VEGGIES

MEAL #4

WHAT I ATE

CALORIES	TIME OF DAY

HUNGER BEFORE	HUNGER AFTER

STARS: ❐ PROTEIN ❐ FIBER ❐ GOOD FATS ❐ FRUITS/VEGGIES

MEAL #5

WHAT I ATE

CALORIES	TIME OF DAY

HUNGER BEFORE	HUNGER AFTER

STARS: ❐ PROTEIN ❐ FIBER ❐ GOOD FATS ❐ FRUITS/VEGGIES

PHYSICAL ACTIVITY

Activity:
Duration:
Intensity:
Calories Burned:

Activity:
Duration:
Intensity:
Calories Burned:

OTHER NOTES

TOTAL CALORIES FOR THE DAY:

TOTAL STARS FOR THE DAY:

Protein
❐ ❐ ❐ ❐ ❐
_____
Fiber
❐ ❐ ❐ ❐ ❐
_____
Good Fats
❐ ❐ ❐ ❐ ❐
_____
Fruits/Veggies
❐ ❐ ❐ ❐ ❐

date:

weight:

MEAL #1

WHAT I ATE

CALORIES | TIME OF DAY

HUNGER BEFORE | HUNGER AFTER

STARS: ☐ PROTEIN ☐ FIBER ☐ GOOD FATS ☐ FRUITS/VEGGIES

MEAL #2

WHAT I ATE

CALORIES | TIME OF DAY

HUNGER BEFORE | HUNGER AFTER

STARS: ☐ PROTEIN ☐ FIBER ☐ GOOD FATS ☐ FRUITS/VEGGIES

MEAL #3

WHAT I ATE

CALORIES | TIME OF DAY

HUNGER BEFORE | HUNGER AFTER

STARS: ☐ PROTEIN ☐ FIBER ☐ GOOD FATS ☐ FRUITS/VEGGIES

MEAL #4

WHAT I ATE

CALORIES	TIME OF DAY

HUNGER BEFORE	HUNGER AFTER

STARS: ☐ PROTEIN ☐ FIBER ☐ GOOD FATS ☐ FRUITS/VEGGIES

MEAL #5

WHAT I ATE

CALORIES	TIME OF DAY

HUNGER BEFORE	HUNGER AFTER

STARS: ☐ PROTEIN ☐ FIBER ☐ GOOD FATS ☐ FRUITS/VEGGIES

PHYSICAL ACTIVITY

Activity:
Duration:
Intensity:
Calories Burned:

Activity:
Duration:
Intensity:
Calories Burned:

OTHER NOTES

TOTAL CALORIES FOR THE DAY:

TOTAL STARS FOR THE DAY:

Protein
☐ ☐ ☐ ☐ ☐
_____

Fiber
☐ ☐ ☐ ☐ ☐
_____

Good Fats
☐ ☐ ☐ ☐ ☐
_____

Fruits/Veggies
☐ ☐ ☐ ☐ ☐

date:

weight:

MEAL #1

WHAT I ATE

CALORIES

TIME
OF DAY

HUNGER
BEFORE

HUNGER
AFTER

STARS: ☐ PROTEIN ☐ FIBER ☐ GOOD FATS ☐ FRUITS/VEGGIES

MEAL #2

WHAT I ATE

CALORIES

TIME
OF DAY

HUNGER
BEFORE

HUNGER
AFTER

STARS: ☐ PROTEIN ☐ FIBER ☐ GOOD FATS ☐ FRUITS/VEGGIES

MEAL #3

WHAT I ATE

CALORIES

TIME
OF DAY

HUNGER
BEFORE

HUNGER
AFTER

STARS: ☐ PROTEIN ☐ FIBER ☐ GOOD FATS ☐ FRUITS/VEGGIES

MEAL #4

WHAT I ATE

CALORIES	TIME OF DAY

HUNGER BEFORE	HUNGER AFTER

STARS: ☐ PROTEIN ☐ FIBER ☐ GOOD FATS ☐ FRUITS/VEGGIES

MEAL #5

WHAT I ATE

CALORIES	TIME OF DAY

HUNGER BEFORE	HUNGER AFTER

STARS: ☐ PROTEIN ☐ FIBER ☐ GOOD FATS ☐ FRUITS/VEGGIES

PHYSICAL ACTIVITY

Activity:
Duration:
Intensity:
Calories Burned:

Activity:
Duration:
Intensity:
Calories Burned:

OTHER NOTES

TOTAL CALORIES FOR THE DAY:

TOTAL STARS FOR THE DAY:

Protein
☐ ☐ ☐ ☐

Fiber
☐ ☐ ☐ ☐

Good Fats
☐ ☐ ☐ ☐

Fruits/Veggies
☐ ☐ ☐ ☐

date:

weight:

MEAL #1

WHAT I ATE

CALORIES | TIME OF DAY

HUNGER BEFORE | HUNGER AFTER

STARS: ☐ PROTEIN ☐ FIBER ☐ GOOD FATS ☐ FRUITS/VEGGIES

MEAL #2

WHAT I ATE

CALORIES | TIME OF DAY

HUNGER BEFORE | HUNGER AFTER

STARS: ☐ PROTEIN ☐ FIBER ☐ GOOD FATS ☐ FRUITS/VEGGIES

MEAL #3

WHAT I ATE

CALORIES | TIME OF DAY

HUNGER BEFORE | HUNGER AFTER

STARS: ☐ PROTEIN ☐ FIBER ☐ GOOD FATS ☐ FRUITS/VEGGIES

MEAL #4

WHAT I ATE

CALORIES	TIME OF DAY
HUNGER BEFORE	HUNGER AFTER

STARS: ☐ PROTEIN ☐ FIBER ☐ GOOD FATS ☐ FRUITS/VEGGIES

MEAL #5

WHAT I ATE

CALORIES	TIME OF DAY
HUNGER BEFORE	HUNGER AFTER

STARS: ☐ PROTEIN ☐ FIBER ☐ GOOD FATS ☐ FRUITS/VEGGIES

PHYSICAL ACTIVITY

Activity:
Duration:
Intensity:
Calories Burned:

Activity:
Duration:
Intensity:
Calories Burned:

OTHER NOTES

TOTAL CALORIES FOR THE DAY:

TOTAL STARS FOR THE DAY:

Protein
☐ ☐ ☐ ☐
_____

Fiber
☐ ☐ ☐ ☐
_____

Good Fats
☐ ☐ ☐ ☐
_____

Fruits/Veggies
☐ ☐ ☐ ☐

date:

weight:

MEAL #1

WHAT I ATE

CALORIES

TIME OF DAY

HUNGER BEFORE

HUNGER AFTER

STARS: ☐ PROTEIN ☐ FIBER ☐ GOOD FATS ☐ FRUITS/VEGGIES

MEAL #2

WHAT I ATE

CALORIES

TIME OF DAY

HUNGER BEFORE

HUNGER AFTER

STARS: ☐ PROTEIN ☐ FIBER ☐ GOOD FATS ☐ FRUITS/VEGGIES

MEAL #3

WHAT I ATE

CALORIES

TIME OF DAY

HUNGER BEFORE

HUNGER AFTER

STARS: ☐ PROTEIN ☐ FIBER ☐ GOOD FATS ☐ FRUITS/VEGGIES

MEAL #4

WHAT I ATE

CALORIES	TIME OF DAY

HUNGER BEFORE	HUNGER AFTER

STARS: ☐ PROTEIN ☐ FIBER ☐ GOOD FATS ☐ FRUITS/VEGGIES

MEAL #5

WHAT I ATE

CALORIES	TIME OF DAY

HUNGER BEFORE	HUNGER AFTER

STARS: ☐ PROTEIN ☐ FIBER ☐ GOOD FATS ☐ FRUITS/VEGGIES

PHYSICAL ACTIVITY

Activity:
Duration:
Intensity:
Calories Burned:

Activity:
Duration:
Intensity:
Calories Burned:

OTHER NOTES

TOTAL CALORIES FOR THE DAY:

TOTAL STARS FOR THE DAY:

Protein
☐ ☐ ☐ ☐ ☐

Fiber
☐ ☐ ☐ ☐ ☐

Good Fats
☐ ☐ ☐ ☐ ☐

Fruits/Veggies
☐ ☐ ☐ ☐ ☐

date:

weight:

MEAL #1

WHAT I ATE

CALORIES	TIME OF DAY
HUNGER BEFORE	HUNGER AFTER

STARS: ❑ PROTEIN ❑ FIBER ❑ GOOD FATS ❑ FRUITS/VEGGIES

MEAL #2

WHAT I ATE

CALORIES	TIME OF DAY
HUNGER BEFORE	HUNGER AFTER

STARS: ❑ PROTEIN ❑ FIBER ❑ GOOD FATS ❑ FRUITS/VEGGIES

MEAL #3

WHAT I ATE

CALORIES	TIME OF DAY
HUNGER BEFORE	HUNGER AFTER

STARS: ❑ PROTEIN ❑ FIBER ❑ GOOD FATS ❑ FRUITS/VEGGIES

MEAL #4

WHAT I ATE

CALORIES	TIME OF DAY

HUNGER BEFORE	HUNGER AFTER

STARS: ☐ PROTEIN ☐ FIBER ☐ GOOD FATS ☐ FRUITS/VEGGIES

MEAL #5

WHAT I ATE

CALORIES	TIME OF DAY

HUNGER BEFORE	HUNGER AFTER

STARS: ☐ PROTEIN ☐ FIBER ☐ GOOD FATS ☐ FRUITS/VEGGIES

PHYSICAL ACTIVITY

Activity:
Duration:
Intensity:
Calories Burned:

Activity:
Duration:
Intensity:
Calories Burned:

OTHER NOTES

TOTAL CALORIES FOR THE DAY:

TOTAL STARS FOR THE DAY:

Protein
☐ ☐ ☐ ☐

Fiber
☐ ☐ ☐ ☐

Good Fats
☐ ☐ ☐ ☐

Fruits/Veggies
☐ ☐ ☐ ☐

date:

weight:

MEAL #1

WHAT I ATE

CALORIES

TIME
OF DAY

HUNGER
BEFORE

HUNGER
AFTER

STARS: ☐ PROTEIN ☐ FIBER ☐ GOOD FATS ☐ FRUITS/VEGGIES

MEAL #2

WHAT I ATE

CALORIES

TIME
OF DAY

HUNGER
BEFORE

HUNGER
AFTER

STARS: ☐ PROTEIN ☐ FIBER ☐ GOOD FATS ☐ FRUITS/VEGGIES

MEAL #3

WHAT I ATE

CALORIES

TIME
OF DAY

HUNGER
BEFORE

HUNGER
AFTER

STARS: ☐ PROTEIN ☐ FIBER ☐ GOOD FATS ☐ FRUITS/VEGGIES

MEAL #4

WHAT I ATE

CALORIES

TIME OF DAY

HUNGER BEFORE

HUNGER AFTER

STARS: ☐ PROTEIN ☐ FIBER ☐ GOOD FATS ☐ FRUITS/VEGGIES

MEAL #5

WHAT I ATE

CALORIES

TIME OF DAY

HUNGER BEFORE

HUNGER AFTER

STARS: ☐ PROTEIN ☐ FIBER ☐ GOOD FATS ☐ FRUITS/VEGGIES

PHYSICAL ACTIVITY

Activity:
Duration:
Intensity:
Calories Burned:

Activity:
Duration:
Intensity:
Calories Burned:

OTHER NOTES

TOTAL CALORIES FOR THE DAY:

TOTAL STARS FOR THE DAY:

Protein

☐ ☐ ☐ ☐

Fiber

☐ ☐ ☐ ☐

Good Fats

☐ ☐ ☐ ☐

Fruits/Veggies

☐ ☐ ☐ ☐

date:

weight:

MEAL #1

WHAT I ATE

CALORIES	TIME OF DAY
HUNGER BEFORE	HUNGER AFTER

STARS: ☐ PROTEIN ☐ FIBER ☐ GOOD FATS ☐ FRUITS/VEGGIES

MEAL #2

WHAT I ATE

CALORIES	TIME OF DAY
HUNGER BEFORE	HUNGER AFTER

STARS: ☐ PROTEIN ☐ FIBER ☐ GOOD FATS ☐ FRUITS/VEGGIES

MEAL #3

WHAT I ATE

CALORIES	TIME OF DAY
HUNGER BEFORE	HUNGER AFTER

STARS: ☐ PROTEIN ☐ FIBER ☐ GOOD FATS ☐ FRUITS/VEGGIES

MEAL #4

WHAT I ATE

CALORIES

TIME
OF DAY

HUNGER
BEFORE

HUNGER
AFTER

STARS: ☐ PROTEIN ☐ FIBER ☐ GOOD FATS ☐ FRUITS/VEGGIES

MEAL #5

WHAT I ATE

CALORIES

TIME
OF DAY

HUNGER
BEFORE

HUNGER
AFTER

STARS: ☐ PROTEIN ☐ FIBER ☐ GOOD FATS ☐ FRUITS/VEGGIES

PHYSICAL ACTIVITY

Activity:
Duration:
Intensity:
Calories Burned:

Activity:
Duration:
Intensity:
Calories Burned:

OTHER NOTES

TOTAL
CALORIES
FOR THE DAY:

TOTAL STARS
FOR THE DAY:

Protein

———————

Fiber

———————

Good Fats

———————

Fruits/Veggies

400 CALORIE FIX TRACKER

date:

weight:

MEAL #1

WHAT I ATE	CALORIES	TIME OF DAY
	HUNGER BEFORE	HUNGER AFTER

STARS: ☐ PROTEIN ☐ FIBER ☐ GOOD FATS ☐ FRUITS/VEGGIES

MEAL #2

WHAT I ATE	CALORIES	TIME OF DAY
	HUNGER BEFORE	HUNGER AFTER

STARS: ☐ PROTEIN ☐ FIBER ☐ GOOD FATS ☐ FRUITS/VEGGIES

MEAL #3

WHAT I ATE	CALORIES	TIME OF DAY
	HUNGER BEFORE	HUNGER AFTER

STARS: ☐ PROTEIN ☐ FIBER ☐ GOOD FATS ☐ FRUITS/VEGGIES

MEAL #4

WHAT I ATE

CALORIES	TIME OF DAY
HUNGER BEFORE	HUNGER AFTER

STARS: ☐ PROTEIN ☐ FIBER ☐ GOOD FATS ☐ FRUITS/VEGGIES

MEAL #5

WHAT I ATE

CALORIES	TIME OF DAY
HUNGER BEFORE	HUNGER AFTER

STARS: ☐ PROTEIN ☐ FIBER ☐ GOOD FATS ☐ FRUITS/VEGGIES

PHYSICAL ACTIVITY

Activity:
Duration:
Intensity:
Calories Burned:

Activity:
Duration:
Intensity:
Calories Burned:

OTHER NOTES

TOTAL CALORIES FOR THE DAY:

TOTAL STARS FOR THE DAY:

Protein
☐ ☐ ☐ ☐ ☐
___
Fiber
☐ ☐ ☐ ☐ ☐
___
Good Fats
☐ ☐ ☐ ☐ ☐
___
Fruits/Veggies
☐ ☐ ☐ ☐ ☐

date:

weight:

MEAL #1

WHAT I ATE

CALORIES

TIME OF DAY

HUNGER BEFORE

HUNGER AFTER

STARS: ☐ PROTEIN ☐ FIBER ☐ GOOD FATS ☐ FRUITS/VEGGIES

MEAL #2

WHAT I ATE

CALORIES

TIME OF DAY

HUNGER BEFORE

HUNGER AFTER

STARS: ☐ PROTEIN ☐ FIBER ☐ GOOD FATS ☐ FRUITS/VEGGIES

MEAL #3

WHAT I ATE

CALORIES

TIME OF DAY

HUNGER BEFORE

HUNGER AFTER

STARS: ☐ PROTEIN ☐ FIBER ☐ GOOD FATS ☐ FRUITS/VEGGIES

MEAL #4

WHAT I ATE

CALORIES

TIME OF DAY

HUNGER BEFORE

HUNGER AFTER

STARS: ☐ PROTEIN ☐ FIBER ☐ GOOD FATS ☐ FRUITS/VEGGIES

MEAL #5

WHAT I ATE

CALORIES

TIME OF DAY

HUNGER BEFORE

HUNGER AFTER

STARS: ☐ PROTEIN ☐ FIBER ☐ GOOD FATS ☐ FRUITS/VEGGIES

PHYSICAL ACTIVITY

Activity:
Duration:
Intensity:
Calories Burned:

Activity:
Duration:
Intensity:
Calories Burned:

OTHER NOTES

TOTAL CALORIES FOR THE DAY:

TOTAL STARS FOR THE DAY:

Protein

☐ ☐ ☐ ☐ ☐

Fiber

☐ ☐ ☐ ☐ ☐

Good Fats

☐ ☐ ☐ ☐ ☐

Fruits/Veggies

☐ ☐ ☐ ☐ ☐

date:

weight:

MEAL #1

WHAT I ATE	CALORIES	TIME OF DAY
	HUNGER BEFORE	HUNGER AFTER

STARS: ☐ PROTEIN ☐ FIBER ☐ GOOD FATS ☐ FRUITS/VEGGIES

MEAL #2

WHAT I ATE	CALORIES	TIME OF DAY
	HUNGER BEFORE	HUNGER AFTER

STARS: ☐ PROTEIN ☐ FIBER ☐ GOOD FATS ☐ FRUITS/VEGGIES

MEAL #3

WHAT I ATE	CALORIES	TIME OF DAY
	HUNGER BEFORE	HUNGER AFTER

STARS: ☐ PROTEIN ☐ FIBER ☐ GOOD FATS ☐ FRUITS/VEGGIES

MEAL #4

WHAT I ATE

CALORIES	TIME OF DAY

HUNGER BEFORE	HUNGER AFTER

STARS: ☐ PROTEIN ☐ FIBER ☐ GOOD FATS ☐ FRUITS/VEGGIES

MEAL #5

WHAT I ATE

CALORIES	TIME OF DAY

HUNGER BEFORE	HUNGER AFTER

STARS: ☐ PROTEIN ☐ FIBER ☐ GOOD FATS ☐ FRUITS/VEGGIES

PHYSICAL ACTIVITY

Activity:
Duration:
Intensity:
Calories Burned:

Activity:
Duration:
Intensity:
Calories Burned:

OTHER NOTES

TOTAL CALORIES FOR THE DAY:

TOTAL STARS FOR THE DAY:

Protein
☐ ☐ ☐ ☐ ☐
___

Fiber
☐ ☐ ☐ ☐ ☐
___

Good Fats
☐ ☐ ☐ ☐ ☐
___

Fruits/Veggies
☐ ☐ ☐ ☐ ☐

400 CALORIE FIX TRACKER

date:

weight:

MEAL #1

WHAT I ATE

CALORIES

TIME OF DAY

HUNGER BEFORE

HUNGER AFTER

STARS: ☐ PROTEIN ☐ FIBER ☐ GOOD FATS ☐ FRUITS/VEGGIES

MEAL #2

WHAT I ATE

CALORIES

TIME OF DAY

HUNGER BEFORE

HUNGER AFTER

STARS: ☐ PROTEIN ☐ FIBER ☐ GOOD FATS ☐ FRUITS/VEGGIES

MEAL #3

WHAT I ATE

CALORIES

TIME OF DAY

HUNGER BEFORE

HUNGER AFTER

STARS: ☐ PROTEIN ☐ FIBER ☐ GOOD FATS ☐ FRUITS/VEGGIES

MEAL #4

WHAT I ATE

CALORIES	TIME OF DAY
HUNGER BEFORE	**HUNGER AFTER**

STARS: ☐ PROTEIN ☐ FIBER ☐ GOOD FATS ☐ FRUITS/VEGGIES

MEAL #5

WHAT I ATE

CALORIES	TIME OF DAY
HUNGER BEFORE	**HUNGER AFTER**

STARS: ☐ PROTEIN ☐ FIBER ☐ GOOD FATS ☐ FRUITS/VEGGIES

PHYSICAL ACTIVITY

Activity:
Duration:
Intensity:
Calories Burned:

Activity:
Duration:
Intensity:
Calories Burned:

OTHER NOTES

TOTAL CALORIES FOR THE DAY:

TOTAL STARS FOR THE DAY:

Protein
☐ ☐ ☐ ☐ ☐

Fiber
☐ ☐ ☐ ☐ ☐

Good Fats
☐ ☐ ☐ ☐ ☐

Fruits/Veggies
☐ ☐ ☐ ☐ ☐

400 CALORIE FIX TRACKER

date:

weight:

MEAL #1

WHAT I ATE

CALORIES

TIME OF DAY

HUNGER BEFORE

HUNGER AFTER

STARS: ☐ PROTEIN ☐ FIBER ☐ GOOD FATS ☐ FRUITS/VEGGIES

MEAL #2

WHAT I ATE

CALORIES

TIME OF DAY

HUNGER BEFORE

HUNGER AFTER

STARS: ☐ PROTEIN ☐ FIBER ☐ GOOD FATS ☐ FRUITS/VEGGIES

MEAL #3

WHAT I ATE

CALORIES

TIME OF DAY

HUNGER BEFORE

HUNGER AFTER

STARS: ☐ PROTEIN ☐ FIBER ☐ GOOD FATS ☐ FRUITS/VEGGIES

MEAL #4

WHAT I ATE

CALORIES

TIME OF DAY

HUNGER BEFORE

HUNGER AFTER

STARS: ☐ PROTEIN ☐ FIBER ☐ GOOD FATS ☐ FRUITS/VEGGIES

MEAL #5

WHAT I ATE

CALORIES

TIME OF DAY

HUNGER BEFORE

HUNGER AFTER

STARS: ☐ PROTEIN ☐ FIBER ☐ GOOD FATS ☐ FRUITS/VEGGIES

PHYSICAL ACTIVITY

Activity:
Duration:
Intensity:
Calories Burned:

Activity:
Duration:
Intensity:
Calories Burned:

OTHER NOTES

TOTAL CALORIES FOR THE DAY:

TOTAL STARS FOR THE DAY:

Protein

☐ ☐ ☐ ☐ ☐

Fiber

☐ ☐ ☐ ☐ ☐

Good Fats

☐ ☐ ☐ ☐ ☐

Fruits/Veggies

☐ ☐ ☐ ☐ ☐

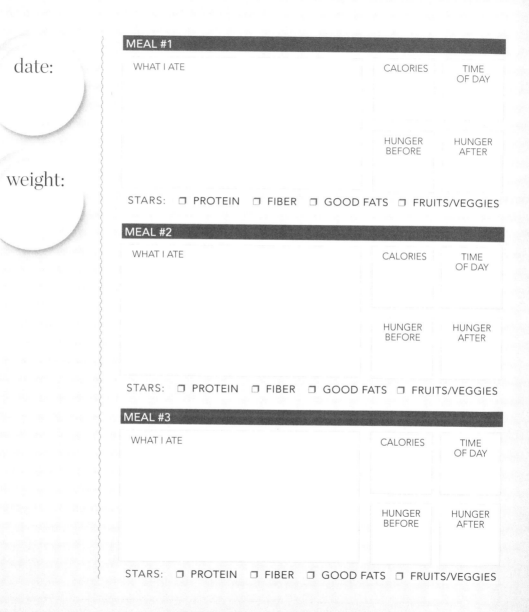

date:

weight:

MEAL #1

WHAT I ATE

CALORIES

TIME OF DAY

HUNGER BEFORE

HUNGER AFTER

STARS: ☐ PROTEIN ☐ FIBER ☐ GOOD FATS ☐ FRUITS/VEGGIES

MEAL #2

WHAT I ATE

CALORIES

TIME OF DAY

HUNGER BEFORE

HUNGER AFTER

STARS: ☐ PROTEIN ☐ FIBER ☐ GOOD FATS ☐ FRUITS/VEGGIES

MEAL #3

WHAT I ATE

CALORIES

TIME OF DAY

HUNGER BEFORE

HUNGER AFTER

STARS: ☐ PROTEIN ☐ FIBER ☐ GOOD FATS ☐ FRUITS/VEGGIES

MEAL #4

WHAT I ATE

CALORIES

TIME OF DAY

HUNGER BEFORE

HUNGER AFTER

STARS: ☐ PROTEIN ☐ FIBER ☐ GOOD FATS ☐ FRUITS/VEGGIES

MEAL #5

WHAT I ATE

CALORIES

TIME OF DAY

HUNGER BEFORE

HUNGER AFTER

STARS: ☐ PROTEIN ☐ FIBER ☐ GOOD FATS ☐ FRUITS/VEGGIES

PHYSICAL ACTIVITY

Activity:
Duration:
Intensity:
Calories Burned:

Activity:
Duration:
Intensity:
Calories Burned:

OTHER NOTES

TOTAL CALORIES FOR THE DAY:

TOTAL STARS FOR THE DAY:

Protein

Fiber

Good Fats

Fruits/Veggies

date:

weight:

MEAL #1

WHAT I ATE

CALORIES

TIME
OF DAY

HUNGER
BEFORE

HUNGER
AFTER

STARS: ☐ PROTEIN ☐ FIBER ☐ GOOD FATS ☐ FRUITS/VEGGIES

MEAL #2

WHAT I ATE

CALORIES

TIME
OF DAY

HUNGER
BEFORE

HUNGER
AFTER

STARS: ☐ PROTEIN ☐ FIBER ☐ GOOD FATS ☐ FRUITS/VEGGIES

MEAL #3

WHAT I ATE

CALORIES

TIME
OF DAY

HUNGER
BEFORE

HUNGER
AFTER

STARS: ☐ PROTEIN ☐ FIBER ☐ GOOD FATS ☐ FRUITS/VEGGIES

MEAL #4

WHAT I ATE

CALORIES	TIME OF DAY
HUNGER BEFORE	HUNGER AFTER

STARS: ☐ PROTEIN ☐ FIBER ☐ GOOD FATS ☐ FRUITS/VEGGIES

MEAL #5

WHAT I ATE

CALORIES	TIME OF DAY
HUNGER BEFORE	HUNGER AFTER

STARS: ☐ PROTEIN ☐ FIBER ☐ GOOD FATS ☐ FRUITS/VEGGIES

PHYSICAL ACTIVITY

Activity:
Duration:
Intensity:
Calories Burned:

Activity:
Duration:
Intensity:
Calories Burned:

OTHER NOTES

TOTAL CALORIES FOR THE DAY:

TOTAL STARS FOR THE DAY:

Protein
☐ ☐ ☐ ☐
_____

Fiber
☐ ☐ ☐ ☐
_____

Good Fats
☐ ☐ ☐ ☐
_____

Fruits/Veggies
☐ ☐ ☐ ☐

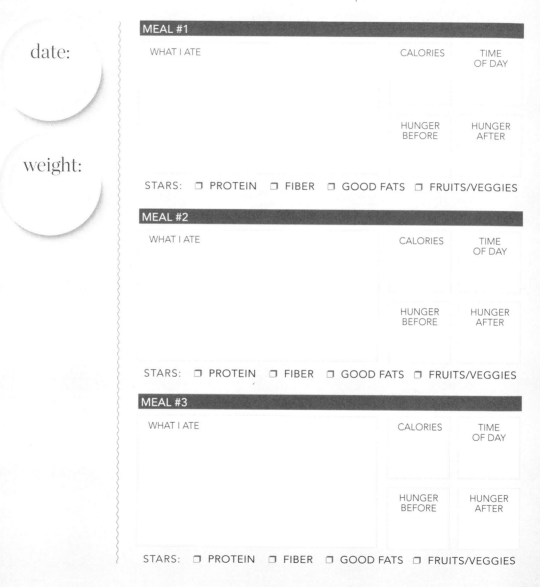

date:

weight:

MEAL #1

WHAT I ATE

CALORIES

TIME OF DAY

HUNGER BEFORE

HUNGER AFTER

STARS: ☐ PROTEIN ☐ FIBER ☐ GOOD FATS ☐ FRUITS/VEGGIES

MEAL #2

WHAT I ATE

CALORIES

TIME OF DAY

HUNGER BEFORE

HUNGER AFTER

STARS: ☐ PROTEIN ☐ FIBER ☐ GOOD FATS ☐ FRUITS/VEGGIES

MEAL #3

WHAT I ATE

CALORIES

TIME OF DAY

HUNGER BEFORE

HUNGER AFTER

STARS: ☐ PROTEIN ☐ FIBER ☐ GOOD FATS ☐ FRUITS/VEGGIES

MEAL #4

WHAT I ATE

CALORIES	TIME OF DAY

HUNGER BEFORE	HUNGER AFTER

STARS: ☐ PROTEIN ☐ FIBER ☐ GOOD FATS ☐ FRUITS/VEGGIES

MEAL #5

WHAT I ATE

CALORIES	TIME OF DAY

HUNGER BEFORE	HUNGER AFTER

STARS: ☐ PROTEIN ☐ FIBER ☐ GOOD FATS ☐ FRUITS/VEGGIES

PHYSICAL ACTIVITY

Activity:
Duration:
Intensity:
Calories Burned:

Activity:
Duration:
Intensity:
Calories Burned:

OTHER NOTES

TOTAL CALORIES FOR THE DAY:

TOTAL STARS FOR THE DAY:

Protein

Fiber

Good Fats

Fruits/Veggies

date:

weight:

MEAL #1

WHAT I ATE

CALORIES   TIME OF DAY

HUNGER BEFORE   HUNGER AFTER

STARS: ☐ PROTEIN ☐ FIBER ☐ GOOD FATS ☐ FRUITS/VEGGIES

MEAL #2

WHAT I ATE

CALORIES   TIME OF DAY

HUNGER BEFORE   HUNGER AFTER

STARS: ☐ PROTEIN ☐ FIBER ☐ GOOD FATS ☐ FRUITS/VEGGIES

MEAL #3

WHAT I ATE

CALORIES   TIME OF DAY

HUNGER BEFORE   HUNGER AFTER

STARS: ☐ PROTEIN ☐ FIBER ☐ GOOD FATS ☐ FRUITS/VEGGIES

MEAL #4

WHAT I ATE

CALORIES	TIME OF DAY

HUNGER BEFORE	HUNGER AFTER

STARS: ☐ PROTEIN ☐ FIBER ☐ GOOD FATS ☐ FRUITS/VEGGIES

MEAL #5

WHAT I ATE

CALORIES	TIME OF DAY

HUNGER BEFORE	HUNGER AFTER

STARS: ☐ PROTEIN ☐ FIBER ☐ GOOD FATS ☐ FRUITS/VEGGIES

PHYSICAL ACTIVITY

Activity:
Duration:
Intensity:
Calories Burned:

Activity:
Duration:
Intensity:
Calories Burned:

OTHER NOTES

TOTAL CALORIES FOR THE DAY:

TOTAL STARS FOR THE DAY:

Protein
☐ ☐ ☐ ☐

Fiber
☐ ☐ ☐ ☐

Good Fats
☐ ☐ ☐ ☐

Fruits/Veggies
☐ ☐ ☐ ☐

date:

weight:

MEAL #1

WHAT I ATE

CALORIES   TIME OF DAY

HUNGER BEFORE   HUNGER AFTER

STARS: ☐ PROTEIN ☐ FIBER ☐ GOOD FATS ☐ FRUITS/VEGGIES

MEAL #2

WHAT I ATE

CALORIES   TIME OF DAY

HUNGER BEFORE   HUNGER AFTER

STARS: ☐ PROTEIN ☐ FIBER ☐ GOOD FATS ☐ FRUITS/VEGGIES

MEAL #3

WHAT I ATE

CALORIES   TIME OF DAY

HUNGER BEFORE   HUNGER AFTER

STARS: ☐ PROTEIN ☐ FIBER ☐ GOOD FATS ☐ FRUITS/VEGGIES

MEAL #4

WHAT I ATE

CALORIES	TIME OF DAY

HUNGER BEFORE	HUNGER AFTER

STARS: ☐ PROTEIN ☐ FIBER ☐ GOOD FATS ☐ FRUITS/VEGGIES

MEAL #5

WHAT I ATE

CALORIES	TIME OF DAY

HUNGER BEFORE	HUNGER AFTER

STARS: ☐ PROTEIN ☐ FIBER ☐ GOOD FATS ☐ FRUITS/VEGGIES

PHYSICAL ACTIVITY

Activity:
Duration:
Intensity:
Calories Burned:

Activity:
Duration:
Intensity:
Calories Burned:

OTHER NOTES

TOTAL CALORIES FOR THE DAY:

TOTAL STARS FOR THE DAY:

Protein
☐ ☐ ☐ ☐

Fiber
☐ ☐ ☐ ☐

Good Fats
☐ ☐ ☐ ☐

Fruits/Veggies
☐ ☐ ☐ ☐

date:

weight:

MEAL #1

WHAT I ATE

CALORIES | TIME OF DAY

HUNGER BEFORE | HUNGER AFTER

STARS: ☐ PROTEIN ☐ FIBER ☐ GOOD FATS ☐ FRUITS/VEGGIES

MEAL #2

WHAT I ATE

CALORIES | TIME OF DAY

HUNGER BEFORE | HUNGER AFTER

STARS: ☐ PROTEIN ☐ FIBER ☐ GOOD FATS ☐ FRUITS/VEGGIES

MEAL #3

WHAT I ATE

CALORIES | TIME OF DAY

HUNGER BEFORE | HUNGER AFTER

STARS: ☐ PROTEIN ☐ FIBER ☐ GOOD FATS ☐ FRUITS/VEGGIES

MEAL #4

WHAT I ATE

CALORIES	TIME OF DAY

HUNGER BEFORE	HUNGER AFTER

STARS: ☐ PROTEIN ☐ FIBER ☐ GOOD FATS ☐ FRUITS/VEGGIES

MEAL #5

WHAT I ATE

CALORIES	TIME OF DAY

HUNGER BEFORE	HUNGER AFTER

STARS: ☐ PROTEIN ☐ FIBER ☐ GOOD FATS ☐ FRUITS/VEGGIES

PHYSICAL ACTIVITY

Activity:
Duration:
Intensity:
Calories Burned:

Activity:
Duration:
Intensity:
Calories Burned:

OTHER NOTES

TOTAL CALORIES FOR THE DAY:

TOTAL STARS FOR THE DAY:

Protein

Fiber

Good Fats

Fruits/Veggies

date:

weight:

MEAL #1

WHAT I ATE

CALORIES

TIME
OF DAY

HUNGER
BEFORE

HUNGER
AFTER

STARS: ☐ PROTEIN ☐ FIBER ☐ GOOD FATS ☐ FRUITS/VEGGIES

MEAL #2

WHAT I ATE

CALORIES

TIME
OF DAY

HUNGER
BEFORE

HUNGER
AFTER

STARS: ☐ PROTEIN ☐ FIBER ☐ GOOD FATS ☐ FRUITS/VEGGIES

MEAL #3

WHAT I ATE

CALORIES

TIME
OF DAY

HUNGER
BEFORE

HUNGER
AFTER

STARS: ☐ PROTEIN ☐ FIBER ☐ GOOD FATS ☐ FRUITS/VEGGIES

MEAL #4

WHAT I ATE

CALORIES	TIME OF DAY

HUNGER BEFORE	HUNGER AFTER

STARS: ☐ PROTEIN ☐ FIBER ☐ GOOD FATS ☐ FRUITS/VEGGIES

MEAL #5

WHAT I ATE

CALORIES	TIME OF DAY

HUNGER BEFORE	HUNGER AFTER

STARS: ☐ PROTEIN ☐ FIBER ☐ GOOD FATS ☐ FRUITS/VEGGIES

PHYSICAL ACTIVITY

Activity:
Duration:
Intensity:
Calories Burned:

Activity:
Duration:
Intensity:
Calories Burned:

OTHER NOTES

TOTAL CALORIES FOR THE DAY:

TOTAL STARS FOR THE DAY:

Protein
☐ ☐ ☐ ☐ ☐

Fiber
☐ ☐ ☐ ☐ ☐

Good Fats
☐ ☐ ☐ ☐ ☐

Fruits/Veggies
☐ ☐ ☐ ☐ ☐

date:

weight:

MEAL #1

WHAT I ATE

CALORIES

TIME
OF DAY

HUNGER
BEFORE

HUNGER
AFTER

STARS: ☐ PROTEIN ☐ FIBER ☐ GOOD FATS ☐ FRUITS/VEGGIES

MEAL #2

WHAT I ATE

CALORIES

TIME
OF DAY

HUNGER
BEFORE

HUNGER
AFTER

STARS: ☐ PROTEIN ☐ FIBER ☐ GOOD FATS ☐ FRUITS/VEGGIES

MEAL #3

WHAT I ATE

CALORIES

TIME
OF DAY

HUNGER
BEFORE

HUNGER
AFTER

STARS: ☐ PROTEIN ☐ FIBER ☐ GOOD FATS ☐ FRUITS/VEGGIES

MEAL #4

WHAT I ATE

CALORIES	TIME OF DAY

HUNGER BEFORE	HUNGER AFTER

STARS: ❑ PROTEIN ❑ FIBER ❑ GOOD FATS ❑ FRUITS/VEGGIES

MEAL #5

WHAT I ATE

CALORIES	TIME OF DAY

HUNGER BEFORE	HUNGER AFTER

STARS: ❑ PROTEIN ❑ FIBER ❑ GOOD FATS ❑ FRUITS/VEGGIES

PHYSICAL ACTIVITY

Activity:
Duration:
Intensity:
Calories Burned:

Activity:
Duration:
Intensity:
Calories Burned:

OTHER NOTES

TOTAL CALORIES FOR THE DAY:

TOTAL STARS FOR THE DAY:

Protein
❑ ❑ ❑ ❑

Fiber
❑ ❑ ❑ ❑

Good Fats
❑ ❑ ❑ ❑

Fruits/Veggies
❑ ❑ ❑ ❑

date:

weight:

MEAL #1

WHAT I ATE

CALORIES

TIME OF DAY

HUNGER BEFORE

HUNGER AFTER

STARS: ☐ PROTEIN ☐ FIBER ☐ GOOD FATS ☐ FRUITS/VEGGIES

MEAL #2

WHAT I ATE

CALORIES

TIME OF DAY

HUNGER BEFORE

HUNGER AFTER

STARS: ☐ PROTEIN ☐ FIBER ☐ GOOD FATS ☐ FRUITS/VEGGIES

MEAL #3

WHAT I ATE

CALORIES

TIME OF DAY

HUNGER BEFORE

HUNGER AFTER

STARS: ☐ PROTEIN ☐ FIBER ☐ GOOD FATS ☐ FRUITS/VEGGIES

MEAL #4

WHAT I ATE

CALORIES	TIME OF DAY
HUNGER BEFORE	HUNGER AFTER

STARS: ☐ PROTEIN ☐ FIBER ☐ GOOD FATS ☐ FRUITS/VEGGIES

MEAL #5

WHAT I ATE

CALORIES	TIME OF DAY
HUNGER BEFORE	HUNGER AFTER

STARS: ☐ PROTEIN ☐ FIBER ☐ GOOD FATS ☐ FRUITS/VEGGIES

PHYSICAL ACTIVITY

Activity:
Duration:
Intensity:
Calories Burned:

Activity:
Duration:
Intensity:
Calories Burned:

OTHER NOTES

TOTAL CALORIES FOR THE DAY:

TOTAL STARS FOR THE DAY:

Protein
☐ ☐ ☐ ☐ ☐

Fiber
☐ ☐ ☐ ☐ ☐

Good Fats
☐ ☐ ☐ ☐ ☐

Fruits/Veggies
☐ ☐ ☐ ☐ ☐

date:

weight:

MEAL #1

WHAT I ATE

CALORIES

TIME OF DAY

HUNGER BEFORE

HUNGER AFTER

STARS: ☐ PROTEIN ☐ FIBER ☐ GOOD FATS ☐ FRUITS/VEGGIES

MEAL #2

WHAT I ATE

CALORIES

TIME OF DAY

HUNGER BEFORE

HUNGER AFTER

STARS: ☐ PROTEIN ☐ FIBER ☐ GOOD FATS ☐ FRUITS/VEGGIES

MEAL #3

WHAT I ATE

CALORIES

TIME OF DAY

HUNGER BEFORE

HUNGER AFTER

STARS: ☐ PROTEIN ☐ FIBER ☐ GOOD FATS ☐ FRUITS/VEGGIES

MEAL #4

WHAT I ATE

CALORIES	TIME OF DAY
HUNGER BEFORE	HUNGER AFTER

STARS: ☐ PROTEIN ☐ FIBER ☐ GOOD FATS ☐ FRUITS/VEGGIES

MEAL #5

WHAT I ATE

CALORIES	TIME OF DAY
HUNGER BEFORE	HUNGER AFTER

STARS: ☐ PROTEIN ☐ FIBER ☐ GOOD FATS ☐ FRUITS/VEGGIES

PHYSICAL ACTIVITY

Activity:
Duration:
Intensity:
Calories Burned:

Activity:
Duration:
Intensity:
Calories Burned:

OTHER NOTES

TOTAL CALORIES FOR THE DAY:

TOTAL STARS FOR THE DAY:

Protein
☐ ☐ ☐ ☐ ☐

Fiber
☐ ☐ ☐ ☐ ☐

Good Fats
☐ ☐ ☐ ☐ ☐

Fruits/Veggies
☐ ☐ ☐ ☐ ☐

date:

weight:

MEAL #1

WHAT I ATE

CALORIES	TIME OF DAY
HUNGER BEFORE	HUNGER AFTER

STARS: ☐ PROTEIN ☐ FIBER ☐ GOOD FATS ☐ FRUITS/VEGGIES

MEAL #2

WHAT I ATE

CALORIES	TIME OF DAY
HUNGER BEFORE	HUNGER AFTER

STARS: ☐ PROTEIN ☐ FIBER ☐ GOOD FATS ☐ FRUITS/VEGGIES

MEAL #3

WHAT I ATE

CALORIES	TIME OF DAY
HUNGER BEFORE	HUNGER AFTER

STARS: ☐ PROTEIN ☐ FIBER ☐ GOOD FATS ☐ FRUITS/VEGGIES

MEAL #4

WHAT I ATE	CALORIES	TIME OF DAY
	HUNGER BEFORE	HUNGER AFTER

STARS: ☐ PROTEIN ☐ FIBER ☐ GOOD FATS ☐ FRUITS/VEGGIES

MEAL #5

WHAT I ATE	CALORIES	TIME OF DAY
	HUNGER BEFORE	HUNGER AFTER

STARS: ☐ PROTEIN ☐ FIBER ☐ GOOD FATS ☐ FRUITS/VEGGIES

PHYSICAL ACTIVITY

Activity:
Duration:
Intensity:
Calories Burned:

Activity:
Duration:
Intensity:
Calories Burned:

OTHER NOTES

TOTAL CALORIES FOR THE DAY:

TOTAL STARS FOR THE DAY:

Protein
ᆨ ᆨ ᆨ ᆨ ᆨ
―――――――
Fiber
ᆨ ᆨ ᆨ ᆨ ᆨ
―――――――
Good Fats
ᆨ ᆨ ᆨ ᆨ ᆨ
―――――――
Fruits/Veggies
ᆨ ᆨ ᆨ ᆨ ᆨ

date:

weight:

MEAL #1

WHAT I ATE	CALORIES	TIME OF DAY
	HUNGER BEFORE	HUNGER AFTER

STARS: ☐ PROTEIN ☐ FIBER ☐ GOOD FATS ☐ FRUITS/VEGGIES

MEAL #2

WHAT I ATE	CALORIES	TIME OF DAY
	HUNGER BEFORE	HUNGER AFTER

STARS: ☐ PROTEIN ☐ FIBER ☐ GOOD FATS ☐ FRUITS/VEGGIES

MEAL #3

WHAT I ATE	CALORIES	TIME OF DAY
	HUNGER BEFORE	HUNGER AFTER

STARS: ☐ PROTEIN ☐ FIBER ☐ GOOD FATS ☐ FRUITS/VEGGIES

MEAL #4

WHAT I ATE

CALORIES	TIME OF DAY
HUNGER BEFORE	HUNGER AFTER

STARS: ☐ PROTEIN ☐ FIBER ☐ GOOD FATS ☐ FRUITS/VEGGIES

MEAL #5

WHAT I ATE

CALORIES	TIME OF DAY
HUNGER BEFORE	HUNGER AFTER

STARS: ☐ PROTEIN ☐ FIBER ☐ GOOD FATS ☐ FRUITS/VEGGIES

PHYSICAL ACTIVITY

Activity:
Duration:
Intensity:
Calories Burned:

Activity:
Duration:
Intensity:
Calories Burned:

OTHER NOTES

TOTAL CALORIES FOR THE DAY:

TOTAL STARS FOR THE DAY:

Protein
☐ ☐ ☐ ☐ ☐

Fiber
☐ ☐ ☐ ☐ ☐

Good Fats
☐ ☐ ☐ ☐ ☐

Fruits/Veggies
☐ ☐ ☐ ☐ ☐

date:

weight:

MEAL #1

WHAT I ATE

CALORIES	TIME OF DAY
HUNGER BEFORE	HUNGER AFTER

STARS: ☐ PROTEIN ☐ FIBER ☐ GOOD FATS ☐ FRUITS/VEGGIES

MEAL #2

WHAT I ATE

CALORIES	TIME OF DAY
HUNGER BEFORE	HUNGER AFTER

STARS: ☐ PROTEIN ☐ FIBER ☐ GOOD FATS ☐ FRUITS/VEGGIES

MEAL #3

WHAT I ATE

CALORIES	TIME OF DAY
HUNGER BEFORE	HUNGER AFTER

STARS: ☐ PROTEIN ☐ FIBER ☐ GOOD FATS ☐ FRUITS/VEGGIES

MEAL #4

WHAT I ATE

CALORIES	TIME OF DAY

HUNGER BEFORE	HUNGER AFTER

STARS: ☐ PROTEIN ☐ FIBER ☐ GOOD FATS ☐ FRUITS/VEGGIES

MEAL #5

WHAT I ATE

CALORIES	TIME OF DAY

HUNGER BEFORE	HUNGER AFTER

STARS: ☐ PROTEIN ☐ FIBER ☐ GOOD FATS ☐ FRUITS/VEGGIES

PHYSICAL ACTIVITY

Activity:
Duration:
Intensity:
Calories Burned:

Activity:
Duration:
Intensity:
Calories Burned:

OTHER NOTES

TOTAL CALORIES FOR THE DAY:

TOTAL STARS FOR THE DAY:

Protein
☐ ☐ ☐ ☐
_____
Fiber
☐ ☐ ☐ ☐
_____
Good Fats
☐ ☐ ☐ ☐
_____
Fruits/Veggies
☐ ☐ ☐ ☐

400 CALORIE FIX TRACKER

date:

weight:

MEAL #1

WHAT I ATE

CALORIES

TIME OF DAY

HUNGER BEFORE

HUNGER AFTER

STARS: ☐ PROTEIN ☐ FIBER ☐ GOOD FATS ☐ FRUITS/VEGGIES

MEAL #2

WHAT I ATE

CALORIES

TIME OF DAY

HUNGER BEFORE

HUNGER AFTER

STARS: ☐ PROTEIN ☐ FIBER ☐ GOOD FATS ☐ FRUITS/VEGGIES

MEAL #3

WHAT I ATE

CALORIES

TIME OF DAY

HUNGER BEFORE

HUNGER AFTER

STARS: ☐ PROTEIN ☐ FIBER ☐ GOOD FATS ☐ FRUITS/VEGGIES

MEAL #4

WHAT I ATE

CALORIES	TIME OF DAY

HUNGER BEFORE	HUNGER AFTER

STARS: ☐ PROTEIN   ☐ FIBER   ☐ GOOD FATS   ☐ FRUITS/VEGGIES

MEAL #5

WHAT I ATE

CALORIES	TIME OF DAY

HUNGER BEFORE	HUNGER AFTER

STARS: ☐ PROTEIN   ☐ FIBER   ☐ GOOD FATS   ☐ FRUITS/VEGGIES

PHYSICAL ACTIVITY

Activity:
Duration:
Intensity:
Calories Burned:

Activity:
Duration:
Intensity:
Calories Burned:

OTHER NOTES

TOTAL CALORIES FOR THE DAY:

TOTAL STARS FOR THE DAY:

Protein

☐ ☐ ☐ ☐ ☐

Fiber

☐ ☐ ☐ ☐ ☐

Good Fats

☐ ☐ ☐ ☐ ☐

Fruits/Veggies

☐ ☐ ☐ ☐ ☐

date:

weight:

MEAL #1

WHAT I ATE

CALORIES	TIME OF DAY
HUNGER BEFORE	HUNGER AFTER

STARS:　☐ PROTEIN　☐ FIBER　☐ GOOD FATS　☐ FRUITS/VEGGIES

MEAL #2

WHAT I ATE

CALORIES	TIME OF DAY
HUNGER BEFORE	HUNGER AFTER

STARS:　☐ PROTEIN　☐ FIBER　☐ GOOD FATS　☐ FRUITS/VEGGIES

MEAL #3

WHAT I ATE

CALORIES	TIME OF DAY
HUNGER BEFORE	HUNGER AFTER

STARS:　☐ PROTEIN　☐ FIBER　☐ GOOD FATS　☐ FRUITS/VEGGIES

MEAL #4

WHAT I ATE

CALORIES	TIME OF DAY

HUNGER BEFORE	HUNGER AFTER

STARS: ☐ PROTEIN ☐ FIBER ☐ GOOD FATS ☐ FRUITS/VEGGIES

MEAL #5

WHAT I ATE

CALORIES	TIME OF DAY

HUNGER BEFORE	HUNGER AFTER

STARS: ☐ PROTEIN ☐ FIBER ☐ GOOD FATS ☐ FRUITS/VEGGIES

PHYSICAL ACTIVITY

Activity:
Duration:
Intensity:
Calories Burned:

Activity:
Duration:
Intensity:
Calories Burned:

OTHER NOTES

TOTAL CALORIES FOR THE DAY:

TOTAL STARS FOR THE DAY:

Protein
☐ ☐ ☐ ☐
_____

Fiber
☐ ☐ ☐ ☐
_____

Good Fats
☐ ☐ ☐ ☐
_____

Fruits/Veggies
☐ ☐ ☐ ☐

date:

weight:

MEAL #1

WHAT I ATE

CALORIES

TIME OF DAY

HUNGER BEFORE

HUNGER AFTER

STARS: ☐ PROTEIN ☐ FIBER ☐ GOOD FATS ☐ FRUITS/VEGGIES

MEAL #2

WHAT I ATE

CALORIES

TIME OF DAY

HUNGER BEFORE

HUNGER AFTER

STARS: ☐ PROTEIN ☐ FIBER ☐ GOOD FATS ☐ FRUITS/VEGGIES

MEAL #3

WHAT I ATE

CALORIES

TIME OF DAY

HUNGER BEFORE

HUNGER AFTER

STARS: ☐ PROTEIN ☐ FIBER ☐ GOOD FATS ☐ FRUITS/VEGGIES

MEAL #4

WHAT I ATE

CALORIES	TIME OF DAY

HUNGER BEFORE	HUNGER AFTER

STARS: ☐ PROTEIN ☐ FIBER ☐ GOOD FATS ☐ FRUITS/VEGGIES

MEAL #5

WHAT I ATE

CALORIES	TIME OF DAY

HUNGER BEFORE	HUNGER AFTER

STARS: ☐ PROTEIN ☐ FIBER ☐ GOOD FATS ☐ FRUITS/VEGGIES

PHYSICAL ACTIVITY

Activity:
Duration:
Intensity:
Calories Burned:

Activity:
Duration:
Intensity:
Calories Burned:

OTHER NOTES

TOTAL CALORIES FOR THE DAY:

TOTAL STARS FOR THE DAY:

Protein
☐ ☐ ☐ ☐ ☐

Fiber
☐ ☐ ☐ ☐ ☐

Good Fats
☐ ☐ ☐ ☐ ☐

Fruits/Veggies
☐ ☐ ☐ ☐ ☐

date:

weight:

MEAL #1

WHAT I ATE

CALORIES	TIME OF DAY
HUNGER BEFORE	HUNGER AFTER

STARS: ☐ PROTEIN   ☐ FIBER   ☐ GOOD FATS   ☐ FRUITS/VEGGIES

MEAL #2

WHAT I ATE

CALORIES	TIME OF DAY
HUNGER BEFORE	HUNGER AFTER

STARS: ☐ PROTEIN   ☐ FIBER   ☐ GOOD FATS   ☐ FRUITS/VEGGIES

MEAL #3

WHAT I ATE

CALORIES	TIME OF DAY
HUNGER BEFORE	HUNGER AFTER

STARS: ☐ PROTEIN   ☐ FIBER   ☐ GOOD FATS   ☐ FRUITS/VEGGIES

MEAL #4

WHAT I ATE

CALORIES	TIME OF DAY

HUNGER BEFORE	HUNGER AFTER

STARS: ☐ PROTEIN ☐ FIBER ☐ GOOD FATS ☐ FRUITS/VEGGIES

MEAL #5

WHAT I ATE

CALORIES	TIME OF DAY

HUNGER BEFORE	HUNGER AFTER

STARS: ☐ PROTEIN ☐ FIBER ☐ GOOD FATS ☐ FRUITS/VEGGIES

PHYSICAL ACTIVITY

Activity:
Duration:
Intensity:
Calories Burned:

Activity:
Duration:
Intensity:
Calories Burned:

OTHER NOTES

TOTAL CALORIES FOR THE DAY:

TOTAL STARS FOR THE DAY:

Protein
❐ ❐ ❐ ❐

Fiber
❐ ❐ ❐ ❐

Good Fats
❐ ❐ ❐ ❐

Fruits/Veggies
❐ ❐ ❐ ❐

date:

weight:

MEAL #1

WHAT I ATE	CALORIES	TIME OF DAY
	HUNGER BEFORE	HUNGER AFTER

STARS: ☐ PROTEIN ☐ FIBER ☐ GOOD FATS ☐ FRUITS/VEGGIES

MEAL #2

WHAT I ATE	CALORIES	TIME OF DAY
	HUNGER BEFORE	HUNGER AFTER

STARS: ☐ PROTEIN ☐ FIBER ☐ GOOD FATS ☐ FRUITS/VEGGIES

MEAL #3

WHAT I ATE	CALORIES	TIME OF DAY
	HUNGER BEFORE	HUNGER AFTER

STARS: ☐ PROTEIN ☐ FIBER ☐ GOOD FATS ☐ FRUITS/VEGGIES

MEAL #4

WHAT I ATE

CALORIES

TIME OF DAY

HUNGER BEFORE

HUNGER AFTER

STARS: ❑ PROTEIN ❑ FIBER ❑ GOOD FATS ❑ FRUITS/VEGGIES

MEAL #5

WHAT I ATE

CALORIES

TIME OF DAY

HUNGER BEFORE

HUNGER AFTER

STARS: ❑ PROTEIN ❑ FIBER ❑ GOOD FATS ❑ FRUITS/VEGGIES

PHYSICAL ACTIVITY

Activity:
Duration:
Intensity:
Calories Burned:

Activity:
Duration:
Intensity:
Calories Burned:

OTHER NOTES

TOTAL CALORIES FOR THE DAY:

TOTAL STARS FOR THE DAY:

Protein
❑ ❑ ❑ ❑

Fiber
❑ ❑ ❑ ❑

Good Fats
❑ ❑ ❑ ❑

Fruits/Veggies
❑ ❑ ❑ ❑

400 CALORIE FIX TRACKER

date:

weight:

MEAL #1

WHAT I ATE

CALORIES	TIME OF DAY
HUNGER BEFORE	HUNGER AFTER

STARS: ❒ PROTEIN ❒ FIBER ❒ GOOD FATS ❒ FRUITS/VEGGIES

MEAL #2

WHAT I ATE

CALORIES	TIME OF DAY
HUNGER BEFORE	HUNGER AFTER

STARS: ❒ PROTEIN ❒ FIBER ❒ GOOD FATS ❒ FRUITS/VEGGIES

MEAL #3

WHAT I ATE

CALORIES	TIME OF DAY
HUNGER BEFORE	HUNGER AFTER

STARS: ❒ PROTEIN ❒ FIBER ❒ GOOD FATS ❒ FRUITS/VEGGIES

MEAL #4

WHAT I ATE

CALORIES	TIME OF DAY

HUNGER BEFORE	HUNGER AFTER

STARS: ☐ PROTEIN ☐ FIBER ☐ GOOD FATS ☐ FRUITS/VEGGIES

MEAL #5

WHAT I ATE

CALORIES	TIME OF DAY

HUNGER BEFORE	HUNGER AFTER

STARS: ☐ PROTEIN ☐ FIBER ☐ GOOD FATS ☐ FRUITS/VEGGIES

PHYSICAL ACTIVITY

Activity:
Duration:
Intensity:
Calories Burned:

Activity:
Duration:
Intensity:
Calories Burned:

OTHER NOTES

TOTAL CALORIES FOR THE DAY:

TOTAL STARS FOR THE DAY:

Protein
☐ ☐ ☐ ☐ ☐
_____

Fiber
☐ ☐ ☐ ☐ ☐
_____

Good Fats
☐ ☐ ☐ ☐ ☐
_____

Fruits/Veggies
☐ ☐ ☐ ☐ ☐

date:

weight:

MEAL #1

WHAT I ATE

CALORIES

TIME OF DAY

HUNGER BEFORE

HUNGER AFTER

STARS: ☐ PROTEIN ☐ FIBER ☐ GOOD FATS ☐ FRUITS/VEGGIES

MEAL #2

WHAT I ATE

CALORIES

TIME OF DAY

HUNGER BEFORE

HUNGER AFTER

STARS: ☐ PROTEIN ☐ FIBER ☐ GOOD FATS ☐ FRUITS/VEGGIES

MEAL #3

WHAT I ATE

CALORIES

TIME OF DAY

HUNGER BEFORE

HUNGER AFTER

STARS: ☐ PROTEIN ☐ FIBER ☐ GOOD FATS ☐ FRUITS/VEGGIES

MEAL #4

WHAT I ATE

CALORIES	TIME OF DAY
HUNGER BEFORE	HUNGER AFTER

STARS: ❐ PROTEIN ❐ FIBER ❐ GOOD FATS ❐ FRUITS/VEGGIES

MEAL #5

WHAT I ATE

CALORIES	TIME OF DAY
HUNGER BEFORE	HUNGER AFTER

STARS: ❐ PROTEIN ❐ FIBER ❐ GOOD FATS ❐ FRUITS/VEGGIES

PHYSICAL ACTIVITY

Activity:
Duration:
Intensity:
Calories Burned:

Activity:
Duration:
Intensity:
Calories Burned:

OTHER NOTES

TOTAL CALORIES FOR THE DAY:

TOTAL STARS FOR THE DAY:

Protein
❐ ❐ ❐ ❐

Fiber
❐ ❐ ❐ ❐

Good Fats
❐ ❐ ❐ ❐

Fruits/Veggies
❐ ❐ ❐ ❐

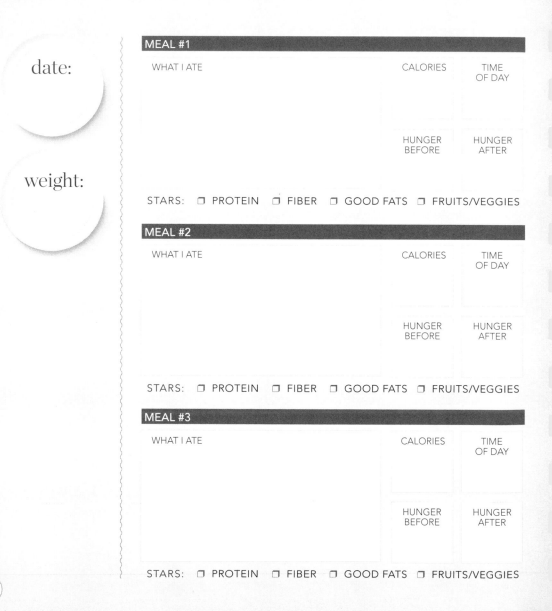

date:

weight:

MEAL #1

WHAT I ATE

CALORIES

TIME OF DAY

HUNGER BEFORE

HUNGER AFTER

STARS: ☐ PROTEIN ☐ FIBER ☐ GOOD FATS ☐ FRUITS/VEGGIES

MEAL #2

WHAT I ATE

CALORIES

TIME OF DAY

HUNGER BEFORE

HUNGER AFTER

STARS: ☐ PROTEIN ☐ FIBER ☐ GOOD FATS ☐ FRUITS/VEGGIES

MEAL #3

WHAT I ATE

CALORIES

TIME OF DAY

HUNGER BEFORE

HUNGER AFTER

STARS: ☐ PROTEIN ☐ FIBER ☐ GOOD FATS ☐ FRUITS/VEGGIES

MEAL #4

WHAT I ATE

CALORIES	TIME OF DAY

HUNGER BEFORE	HUNGER AFTER

STARS: ☐ PROTEIN   ☐ FIBER   ☐ GOOD FATS   ☐ FRUITS/VEGGIES

MEAL #5

WHAT I ATE

CALORIES	TIME OF DAY

HUNGER BEFORE	HUNGER AFTER

STARS: ☐ PROTEIN   ☐ FIBER   ☐ GOOD FATS   ☐ FRUITS/VEGGIES

PHYSICAL ACTIVITY

Activity:
Duration:
Intensity:
Calories Burned:

Activity:
Duration:
Intensity:
Calories Burned:

OTHER NOTES

TOTAL CALORIES FOR THE DAY:

TOTAL STARS FOR THE DAY:

Protein
☐ ☐ ☐ ☐ ☐

Fiber
☐ ☐ ☐ ☐ ☐

Good Fats
☐ ☐ ☐ ☐ ☐

Fruits/Veggies
☐ ☐ ☐ ☐ ☐

date:

weight:

MEAL #1

WHAT I ATE

| CALORIES | TIME OF DAY |
| HUNGER BEFORE | HUNGER AFTER |

STARS: ☐ PROTEIN ☐ FIBER ☐ GOOD FATS ☐ FRUITS/VEGGIES

MEAL #2

WHAT I ATE

| CALORIES | TIME OF DAY |
| HUNGER BEFORE | HUNGER AFTER |

STARS: ☐ PROTEIN ☐ FIBER ☐ GOOD FATS ☐ FRUITS/VEGGIES

MEAL #3

WHAT I ATE

| CALORIES | TIME OF DAY |
| HUNGER BEFORE | HUNGER AFTER |

STARS: ☐ PROTEIN ☐ FIBER ☐ GOOD FATS ☐ FRUITS/VEGGIES

MEAL #4

WHAT I ATE

CALORIES	TIME OF DAY

HUNGER BEFORE	HUNGER AFTER

STARS: ☐ PROTEIN ☐ FIBER ☐ GOOD FATS ☐ FRUITS/VEGGIES

MEAL #5

WHAT I ATE

CALORIES	TIME OF DAY

HUNGER BEFORE	HUNGER AFTER

STARS: ☐ PROTEIN ☐ FIBER ☐ GOOD FATS ☐ FRUITS/VEGGIES

PHYSICAL ACTIVITY

Activity:
Duration:
Intensity:
Calories Burned:

Activity:
Duration:
Intensity:
Calories Burned:

OTHER NOTES

TOTAL CALORIES FOR THE DAY:

TOTAL STARS FOR THE DAY:

Protein
☐ ☐ ☐ ☐ ☐

Fiber
☐ ☐ ☐ ☐ ☐

Good Fats
☐ ☐ ☐ ☐ ☐

Fruits/Veggies
☐ ☐ ☐ ☐

date:

weight:

MEAL #1

WHAT I ATE

| CALORIES | TIME OF DAY |
| HUNGER BEFORE | HUNGER AFTER |

STARS: ❏ PROTEIN   ❏ FIBER   ❏ GOOD FATS   ❏ FRUITS/VEGGIES

MEAL #2

WHAT I ATE

| CALORIES | TIME OF DAY |
| HUNGER BEFORE | HUNGER AFTER |

STARS: ❏ PROTEIN   ❏ FIBER   ❏ GOOD FATS   ❏ FRUITS/VEGGIES

MEAL #3

WHAT I ATE

| CALORIES | TIME OF DAY |
| HUNGER BEFORE | HUNGER AFTER |

STARS: ❏ PROTEIN   ❏ FIBER   ❏ GOOD FATS   ❏ FRUITS/VEGGIES

MEAL #4

WHAT I ATE	CALORIES	TIME OF DAY
	HUNGER BEFORE	HUNGER AFTER

STARS: ☐ PROTEIN   ☐ FIBER   ☐ GOOD FATS   ☐ FRUITS/VEGGIES

MEAL #5

WHAT I ATE	CALORIES	TIME OF DAY
	HUNGER BEFORE	HUNGER AFTER

STARS: ☐ PROTEIN   ☐ FIBER   ☐ GOOD FATS   ☐ FRUITS/VEGGIES

PHYSICAL ACTIVITY

Activity:
Duration:
Intensity:
Calories Burned:

Activity:
Duration:
Intensity:
Calories Burned:

OTHER NOTES

TOTAL CALORIES FOR THE DAY:

TOTAL STARS FOR THE DAY:

Protein
☐ ☐ ☐ ☐ ☐
———
Fiber
☐ ☐ ☐ ☐ ☐
———
Good Fats
☐ ☐ ☐ ☐ ☐
———
Fruits/Veggies
☐ ☐ ☐ ☐ ☐

400 CALORIE FIX TRACKER

date:

weight:

MEAL #1

WHAT I ATE

CALORIES

TIME OF DAY

HUNGER BEFORE

HUNGER AFTER

STARS: ☐ PROTEIN ☐ FIBER ☐ GOOD FATS ☐ FRUITS/VEGGIES

MEAL #2

WHAT I ATE

CALORIES

TIME OF DAY

HUNGER BEFORE

HUNGER AFTER

STARS: ☐ PROTEIN ☐ FIBER ☐ GOOD FATS ☐ FRUITS/VEGGIES

MEAL #3

WHAT I ATE

CALORIES

TIME OF DAY

HUNGER BEFORE

HUNGER AFTER

STARS: ☐ PROTEIN ☐ FIBER ☐ GOOD FATS ☐ FRUITS/VEGGIES

MEAL #4

WHAT I ATE

CALORIES	TIME OF DAY

HUNGER BEFORE	HUNGER AFTER

STARS: ☐ PROTEIN ☐ FIBER ☐ GOOD FATS ☐ FRUITS/VEGGIES

MEAL #5

WHAT I ATE

CALORIES	TIME OF DAY

HUNGER BEFORE	HUNGER AFTER

STARS: ☐ PROTEIN ☐ FIBER ☐ GOOD FATS ☐ FRUITS/VEGGIES

PHYSICAL ACTIVITY

Activity:
Duration:
Intensity:
Calories Burned:

Activity:
Duration:
Intensity:
Calories Burned:

OTHER NOTES

TOTAL CALORIES FOR THE DAY:

TOTAL STARS FOR THE DAY:

Protein

☐ ☐ ☐ ☐

Fiber

☐ ☐ ☐ ☐

Good Fats

☐ ☐ ☐ ☐

Fruits/Veggies

☐ ☐ ☐ ☐

date:

weight:

MEAL #1

WHAT I ATE

CALORIES   TIME
OF DAY

HUNGER   HUNGER
BEFORE   AFTER

STARS: ☐ PROTEIN   ☐ FIBER   ☐ GOOD FATS   ☐ FRUITS/VEGGIES

MEAL #2

WHAT I ATE

CALORIES   TIME
OF DAY

HUNGER   HUNGER
BEFORE   AFTER

STARS: ☐ PROTEIN   ☐ FIBER   ☐ GOOD FATS   ☐ FRUITS/VEGGIES

MEAL #3

WHAT I ATE

CALORIES   TIME
OF DAY

HUNGER   HUNGER
BEFORE   AFTER

STARS: ☐ PROTEIN   ☐ FIBER   ☐ GOOD FATS   ☐ FRUITS/VEGGIES

MEAL #4

WHAT I ATE

CALORIES

TIME OF DAY

HUNGER BEFORE

HUNGER AFTER

STARS: ☐ PROTEIN ☐ FIBER ☐ GOOD FATS ☐ FRUITS/VEGGIES

MEAL #5

WHAT I ATE

CALORIES

TIME OF DAY

HUNGER BEFORE

HUNGER AFTER

STARS: ☐ PROTEIN ☐ FIBER ☐ GOOD FATS ☐ FRUITS/VEGGIES

PHYSICAL ACTIVITY

Activity:
Duration:
Intensity:
Calories Burned:

Activity:
Duration:
Intensity:
Calories Burned:

OTHER NOTES

TOTAL CALORIES FOR THE DAY:

TOTAL STARS FOR THE DAY:

Protein

☐ ☐ ☐ ☐ ☐

Fiber

☐ ☐ ☐ ☐ ☐

Good Fats

☐ ☐ ☐ ☐ ☐

Fruits/Veggies

☐ ☐ ☐ ☐ ☐

date:

weight:

MEAL #1

WHAT I ATE

CALORIES

TIME OF DAY

HUNGER BEFORE

HUNGER AFTER

STARS: ☐ PROTEIN ☐ FIBER ☐ GOOD FATS ☐ FRUITS/VEGGIES

MEAL #2

WHAT I ATE

CALORIES

TIME OF DAY

HUNGER BEFORE

HUNGER AFTER

STARS: ☐ PROTEIN ☐ FIBER ☐ GOOD FATS ☐ FRUITS/VEGGIES

MEAL #3

WHAT I ATE

CALORIES

TIME OF DAY

HUNGER BEFORE

HUNGER AFTER

STARS: ☐ PROTEIN ☐ FIBER ☐ GOOD FATS ☐ FRUITS/VEGGIES

MEAL #4

WHAT I ATE

CALORIES	TIME OF DAY
HUNGER BEFORE	HUNGER AFTER

STARS: ☐ PROTEIN ☐ FIBER ☐ GOOD FATS ☐ FRUITS/VEGGIES

MEAL #5

WHAT I ATE

CALORIES	TIME OF DAY
HUNGER BEFORE	HUNGER AFTER

STARS: ☐ PROTEIN ☐ FIBER ☐ GOOD FATS ☐ FRUITS/VEGGIES

PHYSICAL ACTIVITY

Activity:
Duration:
Intensity:
Calories Burned:

Activity:
Duration:
Intensity:
Calories Burned:

OTHER NOTES

TOTAL CALORIES FOR THE DAY:

TOTAL STARS FOR THE DAY:

Protein
☐ ☐ ☐ ☐ ☐

Fiber
☐ ☐ ☐ ☐ ☐

Good Fats
☐ ☐ ☐ ☐ ☐

Fruits/Veggies
☐ ☐ ☐ ☐ ☐

400 CALORIE FIX TRACKER

date:

weight:

MEAL #1

WHAT I ATE

| CALORIES | TIME OF DAY |

| HUNGER BEFORE | HUNGER AFTER |

STARS: ☐ PROTEIN ☐ FIBER ☐ GOOD FATS ☐ FRUITS/VEGGIES

MEAL #2

WHAT I ATE

| CALORIES | TIME OF DAY |

| HUNGER BEFORE | HUNGER AFTER |

STARS: ☐ PROTEIN ☐ FIBER ☐ GOOD FATS ☐ FRUITS/VEGGIES

MEAL #3

WHAT I ATE

| CALORIES | TIME OF DAY |

| HUNGER BEFORE | HUNGER AFTER |

STARS: ☐ PROTEIN ☐ FIBER ☐ GOOD FATS ☐ FRUITS/VEGGIES

MEAL #4

WHAT I ATE	CALORIES	TIME OF DAY
	HUNGER BEFORE	HUNGER AFTER

STARS: ☐ PROTEIN ☐ FIBER ☐ GOOD FATS ☐ FRUITS/VEGGIES

MEAL #5

WHAT I ATE	CALORIES	TIME OF DAY
	HUNGER BEFORE	HUNGER AFTER

STARS: ☐ PROTEIN ☐ FIBER ☐ GOOD FATS ☐ FRUITS/VEGGIES

PHYSICAL ACTIVITY

Activity:
Duration:
Intensity:
Calories Burned:

Activity:
Duration:
Intensity:
Calories Burned:

OTHER NOTES

TOTAL CALORIES FOR THE DAY:

TOTAL STARS FOR THE DAY:

Protein
☐ ☐ ☐ ☐ ☐

Fiber
☐ ☐ ☐ ☐ ☐

Good Fats
☐ ☐ ☐ ☐ ☐

Fruits/Veggies
☐ ☐ ☐ ☐ ☐

date:

weight:

MEAL #1

WHAT I ATE

CALORIES	TIME OF DAY
HUNGER BEFORE	HUNGER AFTER

STARS: ☐ PROTEIN ☐ FIBER ☐ GOOD FATS ☐ FRUITS/VEGGIES

MEAL #2

WHAT I ATE

CALORIES	TIME OF DAY
HUNGER BEFORE	HUNGER AFTER

STARS: ☐ PROTEIN ☐ FIBER ☐ GOOD FATS ☐ FRUITS/VEGGIES

MEAL #3

WHAT I ATE

CALORIES	TIME OF DAY
HUNGER BEFORE	HUNGER AFTER

STARS: ☐ PROTEIN ☐ FIBER ☐ GOOD FATS ☐ FRUITS/VEGGIES

MEAL #4

WHAT I ATE

CALORIES	TIME OF DAY

HUNGER BEFORE	HUNGER AFTER

STARS: ☐ PROTEIN ☐ FIBER ☐ GOOD FATS ☐ FRUITS/VEGGIES

MEAL #5

WHAT I ATE

CALORIES	TIME OF DAY

HUNGER BEFORE	HUNGER AFTER

STARS: ☐ PROTEIN ☐ FIBER ☐ GOOD FATS ☐ FRUITS/VEGGIES

PHYSICAL ACTIVITY

Activity:
Duration:
Intensity:
Calories Burned:

Activity:
Duration:
Intensity:
Calories Burned:

OTHER NOTES

TOTAL CALORIES FOR THE DAY:

TOTAL STARS FOR THE DAY:

Protein
☐ ☐ ☐ ☐ ☐

Fiber
☐ ☐ ☐ ☐ ☐

Good Fats
☐ ☐ ☐ ☐ ☐

Fruits/Veggies
☐ ☐ ☐ ☐ ☐

400 CALORIE FIX TRACKER

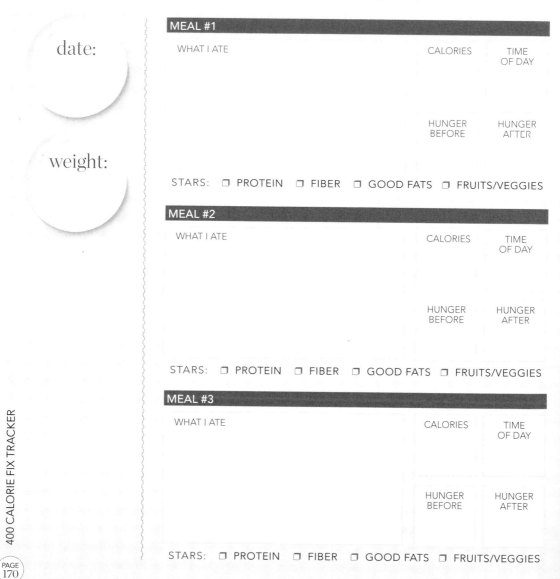

date:

weight:

MEAL #1

WHAT I ATE

CALORIES | TIME OF DAY

HUNGER BEFORE | HUNGER AFTER

STARS: ☐ PROTEIN ☐ FIBER ☐ GOOD FATS ☐ FRUITS/VEGGIES

MEAL #2

WHAT I ATE

CALORIES | TIME OF DAY

HUNGER BEFORE | HUNGER AFTER

STARS: ☐ PROTEIN ☐ FIBER ☐ GOOD FATS ☐ FRUITS/VEGGIES

MEAL #3

WHAT I ATE

CALORIES | TIME OF DAY

HUNGER BEFORE | HUNGER AFTER

STARS: ☐ PROTEIN ☐ FIBER ☐ GOOD FATS ☐ FRUITS/VEGGIES

MEAL #4

WHAT I ATE

CALORIES	TIME OF DAY

HUNGER BEFORE	HUNGER AFTER

STARS: ☐ PROTEIN ☐ FIBER ☐ GOOD FATS ☐ FRUITS/VEGGIES

MEAL #5

WHAT I ATE

CALORIES	TIME OF DAY

HUNGER BEFORE	HUNGER AFTER

STARS: ☐ PROTEIN ☐ FIBER ☐ GOOD FATS ☐ FRUITS/VEGGIES

PHYSICAL ACTIVITY

Activity:
Duration:
Intensity:
Calories Burned:

Activity:
Duration:
Intensity:
Calories Burned:

OTHER NOTES

TOTAL CALORIES FOR THE DAY:

TOTAL STARS FOR THE DAY:

Protein
☐ ☐ ☐ ☐ ☐

Fiber
☐ ☐ ☐ ☐ ☐

Good Fats
☐ ☐ ☐ ☐ ☐

Fruits/Veggies
☐ ☐ ☐ ☐ ☐

date:

weight:

MEAL #1

WHAT I ATE

CALORIES	TIME OF DAY
HUNGER BEFORE	HUNGER AFTER

STARS: ☐ PROTEIN ☐ FIBER ☐ GOOD FATS ☐ FRUITS/VEGGIES

MEAL #2

WHAT I ATE

CALORIES	TIME OF DAY
HUNGER BEFORE	HUNGER AFTER

STARS: ☐ PROTEIN ☐ FIBER ☐ GOOD FATS ☐ FRUITS/VEGGIES

MEAL #3

WHAT I ATE

CALORIES	TIME OF DAY
HUNGER BEFORE	HUNGER AFTER

STARS: ☐ PROTEIN ☐ FIBER ☐ GOOD FATS ☐ FRUITS/VEGGIES

MEAL #4

WHAT I ATE

CALORIES	TIME OF DAY
HUNGER BEFORE	HUNGER AFTER

STARS: ☐ PROTEIN ☐ FIBER ☐ GOOD FATS ☐ FRUITS/VEGGIES

MEAL #5

WHAT I ATE

CALORIES	TIME OF DAY
HUNGER BEFORE	HUNGER AFTER

STARS: ☐ PROTEIN ☐ FIBER ☐ GOOD FATS ☐ FRUITS/VEGGIES

PHYSICAL ACTIVITY

Activity:
Duration:
Intensity:
Calories Burned:

Activity:
Duration:
Intensity:
Calories Burned:

OTHER NOTES

TOTAL CALORIES FOR THE DAY:

TOTAL STARS FOR THE DAY:

Protein
☐ ☐ ☐ ☐ ☐

Fiber
☐ ☐ ☐ ☐ ☐

Good Fats
☐ ☐ ☐ ☐ ☐

Fruits/Veggies
☐ ☐ ☐ ☐ ☐

date:

weight:

MEAL #1

WHAT I ATE

CALORIES

TIME OF DAY

HUNGER BEFORE

HUNGER AFTER

STARS: ☐ PROTEIN ☐ FIBER ☐ GOOD FATS ☐ FRUITS/VEGGIES

MEAL #2

WHAT I ATE

CALORIES

TIME OF DAY

HUNGER BEFORE

HUNGER AFTER

STARS: ☐ PROTEIN ☐ FIBER ☐ GOOD FATS ☐ FRUITS/VEGGIES

MEAL #3

WHAT I ATE

CALORIES

TIME OF DAY

HUNGER BEFORE

HUNGER AFTER

STARS: ☐ PROTEIN ☐ FIBER ☐ GOOD FATS ☐ FRUITS/VEGGIES

MEAL #4

WHAT I ATE	CALORIES	TIME OF DAY
	HUNGER BEFORE	HUNGER AFTER

STARS: ☐ PROTEIN   ☐ FIBER   ☐ GOOD FATS   ☐ FRUITS/VEGGIES

MEAL #5

WHAT I ATE	CALORIES	TIME OF DAY
	HUNGER BEFORE	HUNGER AFTER

STARS: ☐ PROTEIN   ☐ FIBER   ☐ GOOD FATS   ☐ FRUITS/VEGGIES

PHYSICAL ACTIVITY

Activity:
Duration:
Intensity:
Calories Burned:

Activity:
Duration:
Intensity:
Calories Burned:

OTHER NOTES

TOTAL CALORIES FOR THE DAY:

TOTAL STARS FOR THE DAY:

Protein
☐ ☐ ☐ ☐
_____
Fiber
☐ ☐ ☐ ☐
_____
Good Fats
☐ ☐ ☐ ☐
_____
Fruits/Veggies
☐ ☐ ☐ ☐

date:

weight:

MEAL #1

WHAT I ATE

CALORIES

TIME
OF DAY

HUNGER
BEFORE

HUNGER
AFTER

STARS: ☐ PROTEIN   ☐ FIBER   ☐ GOOD FATS   ☐ FRUITS/VEGGIES

MEAL #2

WHAT I ATE

CALORIES

TIME
OF DAY

HUNGER
BEFORE

HUNGER
AFTER

STARS: ☐ PROTEIN   ☐ FIBER   ☐ GOOD FATS   ☐ FRUITS/VEGGIES

MEAL #3

WHAT I ATE

CALORIES

TIME
OF DAY

HUNGER
BEFORE

HUNGER
AFTER

STARS: ☐ PROTEIN   ☐ FIBER   ☐ GOOD FATS   ☐ FRUITS/VEGGIES

MEAL #4

WHAT I ATE

CALORIES	TIME OF DAY
HUNGER BEFORE	HUNGER AFTER

STARS: ☐ PROTEIN ☐ FIBER ☐ GOOD FATS ☐ FRUITS/VEGGIES

MEAL #5

WHAT I ATE

CALORIES	TIME OF DAY
HUNGER BEFORE	HUNGER AFTER

STARS: ☐ PROTEIN ☐ FIBER ☐ GOOD FATS ☐ FRUITS/VEGGIES

PHYSICAL ACTIVITY

Activity:
Duration:
Intensity:
Calories Burned:

Activity:
Duration:
Intensity:
Calories Burned:

OTHER NOTES

TOTAL CALORIES FOR THE DAY:

TOTAL STARS FOR THE DAY:

Protein
☐ ☐ ☐ ☐ ☐

Fiber
☐ ☐ ☐ ☐ ☐

Good Fats
☐ ☐ ☐ ☐ ☐

Fruits/Veggies
☐ ☐ ☐ ☐ ☐

date:

weight:

MEAL #1

WHAT I ATE

CALORIES	TIME OF DAY

HUNGER BEFORE	HUNGER AFTER

STARS: ☐ PROTEIN ☐ FIBER ☐ GOOD FATS ☐ FRUITS/VEGGIES

MEAL #2

WHAT I ATE

CALORIES	TIME OF DAY

HUNGER BEFORE	HUNGER AFTER

STARS: ☐ PROTEIN ☐ FIBER ☐ GOOD FATS ☐ FRUITS/VEGGIES

MEAL #3

WHAT I ATE

CALORIES	TIME OF DAY

HUNGER BEFORE	HUNGER AFTER

STARS: ☐ PROTEIN ☐ FIBER ☐ GOOD FATS ☐ FRUITS/VEGGIES

MEAL #4

WHAT I ATE

CALORIES	TIME OF DAY

HUNGER BEFORE	HUNGER AFTER

STARS: ☐ PROTEIN ☐ FIBER ☐ GOOD FATS ☐ FRUITS/VEGGIES

MEAL #5

WHAT I ATE

CALORIES	TIME OF DAY

HUNGER BEFORE	HUNGER AFTER

STARS: ☐ PROTEIN ☐ FIBER ☐ GOOD FATS ☐ FRUITS/VEGGIES

PHYSICAL ACTIVITY

Activity:
Duration:
Intensity:
Calories Burned:

Activity:
Duration:
Intensity:
Calories Burned:

OTHER NOTES

TOTAL CALORIES FOR THE DAY:

TOTAL STARS FOR THE DAY:

Protein
☐ ☐ ☐ ☐ ☐

Fiber
☐ ☐ ☐ ☐ ☐

Good Fats
☐ ☐ ☐ ☐ ☐

Fruits/Veggies
☐ ☐ ☐ ☐ ☐

date:

weight:

MEAL #1

WHAT I ATE

CALORIES

TIME OF DAY

HUNGER BEFORE

HUNGER AFTER

STARS: ☐ PROTEIN ☐ FIBER ☐ GOOD FATS ☐ FRUITS/VEGGIES

MEAL #2

WHAT I ATE

CALORIES

TIME OF DAY

HUNGER BEFORE

HUNGER AFTER

STARS: ☐ PROTEIN ☐ FIBER ☐ GOOD FATS ☐ FRUITS/VEGGIES

MEAL #3

WHAT I ATE

CALORIES

TIME OF DAY

HUNGER BEFORE

HUNGER AFTER

STARS: ☐ PROTEIN ☐ FIBER ☐ GOOD FATS ☐ FRUITS/VEGGIES

MEAL #4

WHAT I ATE

CALORIES

TIME OF DAY

HUNGER BEFORE

HUNGER AFTER

STARS: ☐ PROTEIN ☐ FIBER ☐ GOOD FATS ☐ FRUITS/VEGGIES

MEAL #5

WHAT I ATE

CALORIES

TIME OF DAY

HUNGER BEFORE

HUNGER AFTER

STARS: ☐ PROTEIN ☐ FIBER ☐ GOOD FATS ☐ FRUITS/VEGGIES

PHYSICAL ACTIVITY

Activity:
Duration:
Intensity:
Calories Burned:

Activity:
Duration:
Intensity:
Calories Burned:

OTHER NOTES

TOTAL CALORIES FOR THE DAY:

TOTAL STARS FOR THE DAY:

Protein

☐ ☐ ☐ ☐ ☐

Fiber

☐ ☐ ☐ ☐ ☐

Good Fats

☐ ☐ ☐ ☐ ☐

Fruits/Veggies

☐ ☐ ☐ ☐ ☐

date:

weight:

MEAL #1

WHAT I ATE

CALORIES

TIME OF DAY

HUNGER BEFORE

HUNGER AFTER

STARS: ☐ PROTEIN ☐ FIBER ☐ GOOD FATS ☐ FRUITS/VEGGIES

MEAL #2

WHAT I ATE

CALORIES

TIME OF DAY

HUNGER BEFORE

HUNGER AFTER

STARS: ☐ PROTEIN ☐ FIBER ☐ GOOD FATS ☐ FRUITS/VEGGIES

MEAL #3

WHAT I ATE

CALORIES

TIME OF DAY

HUNGER BEFORE

HUNGER AFTER

STARS: ☐ PROTEIN ☐ FIBER ☐ GOOD FATS ☐ FRUITS/VEGGIES

MEAL #4

WHAT I ATE

CALORIES

TIME OF DAY

HUNGER BEFORE

HUNGER AFTER

STARS: ☐ PROTEIN ☐ FIBER ☐ GOOD FATS ☐ FRUITS/VEGGIES

MEAL #5

WHAT I ATE

CALORIES

TIME OF DAY

HUNGER BEFORE

HUNGER AFTER

STARS: ☐ PROTEIN ☐ FIBER ☐ GOOD FATS ☐ FRUITS/VEGGIES

PHYSICAL ACTIVITY

Activity:
Duration:
Intensity:
Calories Burned:

Activity:
Duration:
Intensity:
Calories Burned:

OTHER NOTES

TOTAL CALORIES FOR THE DAY:

TOTAL STARS FOR THE DAY:

Protein

☐ ☐ ☐ ☐ ☐

Fiber

☐ ☐ ☐ ☐ ☐

Good Fats

☐ ☐ ☐ ☐ ☐

Fruits/Veggies

☐ ☐ ☐ ☐ ☐

date:

weight:

MEAL #1

WHAT I ATE

CALORIES   TIME
                  OF DAY

HUNGER   HUNGER
BEFORE   AFTER

STARS: ☐ PROTEIN   ☐ FIBER   ☐ GOOD FATS   ☐ FRUITS/VEGGIES

MEAL #2

WHAT I ATE

CALORIES   TIME
                  OF DAY

HUNGER   HUNGER
BEFORE   AFTER

STARS: ☐ PROTEIN   ☐ FIBER   ☐ GOOD FATS   ☐ FRUITS/VEGGIES

MEAL #3

WHAT I ATE

CALORIES   TIME
                  OF DAY

HUNGER   HUNGER
BEFORE   AFTER

STARS: ☐ PROTEIN   ☐ FIBER   ☐ GOOD FATS   ☐ FRUITS/VEGGIES

400 CALORIE FIX TRACKER

MEAL #4

WHAT I ATE

CALORIES	TIME OF DAY

HUNGER BEFORE	HUNGER AFTER

STARS: ☐ PROTEIN ☐ FIBER ☐ GOOD FATS ☐ FRUITS/VEGGIES

MEAL #5

WHAT I ATE

CALORIES	TIME OF DAY

HUNGER BEFORE	HUNGER AFTER

STARS: ☐ PROTEIN ☐ FIBER ☐ GOOD FATS ☐ FRUITS/VEGGIES

PHYSICAL ACTIVITY

Activity:
Duration:
Intensity:
Calories Burned:

Activity:
Duration:
Intensity:
Calories Burned:

OTHER NOTES

TOTAL CALORIES FOR THE DAY:

TOTAL STARS FOR THE DAY:

Protein
☐ ☐ ☐ ☐ ☐

Fiber
☐ ☐ ☐ ☐ ☐

Good Fats
☐ ☐ ☐ ☐ ☐

Fruits/Veggies
☐ ☐ ☐ ☐ ☐

date:

weight:

MEAL #1

WHAT I ATE

CALORIES

TIME
OF DAY

HUNGER
BEFORE

HUNGER
AFTER

STARS: ☐ PROTEIN ☐ FIBER ☐ GOOD FATS ☐ FRUITS/VEGGIES

MEAL #2

WHAT I ATE

CALORIES

TIME
OF DAY

HUNGER
BEFORE

HUNGER
AFTER

STARS: ☐ PROTEIN ☐ FIBER ☐ GOOD FATS ☐ FRUITS/VEGGIES

MEAL #3

WHAT I ATE

CALORIES

TIME
OF DAY

HUNGER
BEFORE

HUNGER
AFTER

STARS: ☐ PROTEIN ☐ FIBER ☐ GOOD FATS ☐ FRUITS/VEGGIES

MEAL #4

WHAT I ATE

CALORIES

TIME OF DAY

HUNGER BEFORE

HUNGER AFTER

STARS: ☐ PROTEIN ☐ FIBER ☐ GOOD FATS ☐ FRUITS/VEGGIES

MEAL #5

WHAT I ATE

CALORIES

TIME OF DAY

HUNGER BEFORE

HUNGER AFTER

STARS: ☐ PROTEIN ☐ FIBER ☐ GOOD FATS ☐ FRUITS/VEGGIES

PHYSICAL ACTIVITY

Activity:
Duration:
Intensity:
Calories Burned:

Activity:
Duration:
Intensity:
Calories Burned:

OTHER NOTES

TOTAL CALORIES FOR THE DAY:

TOTAL STARS FOR THE DAY:

Protein
☐ ☐ ☐ ☐ ☐

Fiber
☐ ☐ ☐ ☐ ☐

Good Fats
☐ ☐ ☐ ☐ ☐

Fruits/Veggies
☐ ☐ ☐ ☐ ☐

date:

weight:

MEAL #1

WHAT I ATE

CALORIES   TIME
OF DAY

HUNGER   HUNGER
BEFORE   AFTER

STARS: ❐ PROTEIN ❐ FIBER ❐ GOOD FATS ❐ FRUITS/VEGGIES

MEAL #2

WHAT I ATE

CALORIES   TIME
OF DAY

HUNGER   HUNGER
BEFORE   AFTER

STARS: ❐ PROTEIN ❐ FIBER ❐ GOOD FATS ❐ FRUITS/VEGGIES

MEAL #3

WHAT I ATE

CALORIES   TIME
OF DAY

HUNGER   HUNGER
BEFORE   AFTER

STARS: ❐ PROTEIN ❐ FIBER ❐ GOOD FATS ❐ FRUITS/VEGGIES

MEAL #4

WHAT I ATE

CALORIES	TIME OF DAY

HUNGER BEFORE	HUNGER AFTER

STARS:　☐ PROTEIN　☐ FIBER　☐ GOOD FATS　☐ FRUITS/VEGGIES

MEAL #5

WHAT I ATE

CALORIES	TIME OF DAY

HUNGER BEFORE	HUNGER AFTER

STARS:　☐ PROTEIN　☐ FIBER　☐ GOOD FATS　☐ FRUITS/VEGGIES

PHYSICAL ACTIVITY

Activity:
Duration:
Intensity:
Calories Burned:

Activity:
Duration:
Intensity:
Calories Burned:

OTHER NOTES

TOTAL CALORIES FOR THE DAY:

TOTAL STARS FOR THE DAY:

Protein
☐ ☐ ☐ ☐ ☐

Fiber
☐ ☐ ☐ ☐ ☐

Good Fats
☐ ☐ ☐ ☐ ☐

Fruits/Veggies
☐ ☐ ☐ ☐ ☐

date:

weight:

MEAL #1

WHAT I ATE

CALORIES

TIME
OF DAY

HUNGER
BEFORE

HUNGER
AFTER

STARS: ❒ PROTEIN   ❒ FIBER   ❒ GOOD FATS   ❒ FRUITS/VEGGIES

MEAL #2

WHAT I ATE

CALORIES

TIME
OF DAY

HUNGER
BEFORE

HUNGER
AFTER

STARS: ❒ PROTEIN   ❒ FIBER   ❒ GOOD FATS   ❒ FRUITS/VEGGIES

MEAL #3

WHAT I ATE

CALORIES

TIME
OF DAY

HUNGER
BEFORE

HUNGER
AFTER

STARS: ❒ PROTEIN   ❒ FIBER   ❒ GOOD FATS   ❒ FRUITS/VEGGIES

MEAL #4

WHAT I ATE

CALORIES	TIME OF DAY

HUNGER BEFORE	HUNGER AFTER

STARS: ☐ PROTEIN ☐ FIBER ☐ GOOD FATS ☐ FRUITS/VEGGIES

MEAL #5

WHAT I ATE

CALORIES	TIME OF DAY

HUNGER BEFORE	HUNGER AFTER

STARS: ☐ PROTEIN ☐ FIBER ☐ GOOD FATS ☐ FRUITS/VEGGIES

PHYSICAL ACTIVITY

Activity:
Duration:
Intensity:
Calories Burned:

Activity:
Duration:
Intensity:
Calories Burned:

OTHER NOTES

TOTAL CALORIES FOR THE DAY:

TOTAL STARS FOR THE DAY:

Protein
☐ ☐ ☐ ☐
_____

Fiber
☐ ☐ ☐ ☐
_____

Good Fats
☐ ☐ ☐ ☐
_____

Fruits/Veggies
☐ ☐ ☐ ☐

date:

weight:

MEAL #1

WHAT I ATE

CALORIES   TIME
OF DAY

HUNGER   HUNGER
BEFORE   AFTER

STARS: ☐ PROTEIN   ☐ FIBER   ☐ GOOD FATS   ☐ FRUITS/VEGGIES

MEAL #2

WHAT I ATE

CALORIES   TIME
OF DAY

HUNGER   HUNGER
BEFORE   AFTER

STARS: ☐ PROTEIN   ☐ FIBER   ☐ GOOD FATS   ☐ FRUITS/VEGGIES

MEAL #3

WHAT I ATE

CALORIES   TIME
OF DAY

HUNGER   HUNGER
BEFORE   AFTER

STARS: ☐ PROTEIN   ☐ FIBER   ☐ GOOD FATS   ☐ FRUITS/VEGGIES

MEAL #4

WHAT I ATE	CALORIES	TIME OF DAY
	HUNGER BEFORE	HUNGER AFTER

STARS: ☐ PROTEIN ☐ FIBER ☐ GOOD FATS ☐ FRUITS/VEGGIES

MEAL #5

WHAT I ATE	CALORIES	TIME OF DAY
	HUNGER BEFORE	HUNGER AFTER

STARS: ☐ PROTEIN ☐ FIBER ☐ GOOD FATS ☐ FRUITS/VEGGIES

PHYSICAL ACTIVITY

Activity:
Duration:
Intensity:
Calories Burned:

Activity:
Duration:
Intensity:
Calories Burned:

OTHER NOTES

TOTAL CALORIES FOR THE DAY:

TOTAL STARS FOR THE DAY:

Protein
☐ ☐ ☐ ☐ ☐

Fiber
☐ ☐ ☐ ☐ ☐

Good Fats
☐ ☐ ☐ ☐ ☐

Fruits/Veggies
☐ ☐ ☐ ☐ ☐

date:

weight:

MEAL #1

WHAT I ATE		CALORIES	TIME OF DAY
		HUNGER BEFORE	HUNGER AFTER

STARS: ☐ PROTEIN   ☐ FIBER   ☐ GOOD FATS   ☐ FRUITS/VEGGIES

MEAL #2

WHAT I ATE		CALORIES	TIME OF DAY
		HUNGER BEFORE	HUNGER AFTER

STARS: ☐ PROTEIN   ☐ FIBER   ☐ GOOD FATS   ☐ FRUITS/VEGGIES

MEAL #3

WHAT I ATE		CALORIES	TIME OF DAY
		HUNGER BEFORE	HUNGER AFTER

STARS: ☐ PROTEIN   ☐ FIBER   ☐ GOOD FATS   ☐ FRUITS/VEGGIES

MEAL #4

WHAT I ATE

CALORIES	TIME OF DAY

HUNGER BEFORE	HUNGER AFTER

STARS: ☐ PROTEIN ☐ FIBER ☐ GOOD FATS ☐ FRUITS/VEGGIES

MEAL #5

WHAT I ATE

CALORIES	TIME OF DAY

HUNGER BEFORE	HUNGER AFTER

STARS: ☐ PROTEIN ☐ FIBER ☐ GOOD FATS ☐ FRUITS/VEGGIES

PHYSICAL ACTIVITY

Activity:
Duration:
Intensity:
Calories Burned:

Activity:
Duration:
Intensity:
Calories Burned:

OTHER NOTES

TOTAL CALORIES FOR THE DAY:

TOTAL STARS FOR THE DAY:

Protein
☐ ☐ ☐ ☐
_____

Fiber
☐ ☐ ☐ ☐
_____

Good Fats
☐ ☐ ☐ ☐
_____

Fruits/Veggies
☐ ☐ ☐ ☐

date:

weight:

MEAL #1

WHAT I ATE

CALORIES

TIME OF DAY

HUNGER BEFORE

HUNGER AFTER

STARS: ☐ PROTEIN ☐ FIBER ☐ GOOD FATS ☐ FRUITS/VEGGIES

MEAL #2

WHAT I ATE

CALORIES

TIME OF DAY

HUNGER BEFORE

HUNGER AFTER

STARS: ☐ PROTEIN ☐ FIBER ☐ GOOD FATS ☐ FRUITS/VEGGIES

MEAL #3

WHAT I ATE

CALORIES

TIME OF DAY

HUNGER BEFORE

HUNGER AFTER

STARS: ☐ PROTEIN ☐ FIBER ☐ GOOD FATS ☐ FRUITS/VEGGIES

MEAL #4

WHAT I ATE

CALORIES	TIME OF DAY
HUNGER BEFORE	HUNGER AFTER

STARS: ☐ PROTEIN ☐ FIBER ☐ GOOD FATS ☐ FRUITS/VEGGIES

MEAL #5

WHAT I ATE

CALORIES	TIME OF DAY
HUNGER BEFORE	HUNGER AFTER

STARS: ☐ PROTEIN ☐ FIBER ☐ GOOD FATS ☐ FRUITS/VEGGIES

PHYSICAL ACTIVITY

Activity:
Duration:
Intensity:
Calories Burned:

Activity:
Duration:
Intensity:
Calories Burned:

OTHER NOTES

TOTAL CALORIES FOR THE DAY:

TOTAL STARS FOR THE DAY:

Protein
☐ ☐ ☐ ☐ ☐

Fiber
☐ ☐ ☐ ☐ ☐

Good Fats
☐ ☐ ☐ ☐ ☐

Fruits/Veggies
☐ ☐ ☐ ☐ ☐

date:

weight:

MEAL #1

WHAT I ATE

CALORIES

TIME OF DAY

HUNGER BEFORE

HUNGER AFTER

STARS: ☐ PROTEIN ☐ FIBER ☐ GOOD FATS ☐ FRUITS/VEGGIES

MEAL #2

WHAT I ATE

CALORIES

TIME OF DAY

HUNGER BEFORE

HUNGER AFTER

STARS: ☐ PROTEIN ☐ FIBER ☐ GOOD FATS ☐ FRUITS/VEGGIES

MEAL #3

WHAT I ATE

CALORIES

TIME OF DAY

HUNGER BEFORE

HUNGER AFTER

STARS: ☐ PROTEIN ☐ FIBER ☐ GOOD FATS ☐ FRUITS/VEGGIES

MEAL #4

WHAT I ATE

CALORIES

TIME OF DAY

HUNGER BEFORE

HUNGER AFTER

STARS: ☐ PROTEIN ☐ FIBER ☐ GOOD FATS ☐ FRUITS/VEGGIES

MEAL #5

WHAT I ATE

CALORIES

TIME OF DAY

HUNGER BEFORE

HUNGER AFTER

STARS: ☐ PROTEIN ☐ FIBER ☐ GOOD FATS ☐ FRUITS/VEGGIES

PHYSICAL ACTIVITY

Activity:
Duration:
Intensity:
Calories Burned:

Activity:
Duration:
Intensity:
Calories Burned:

OTHER NOTES

TOTAL CALORIES FOR THE DAY:

TOTAL STARS FOR THE DAY:

Protein

————————

Fiber

————————

Good Fats

————————

Fruits/Veggies

date:

weight:

MEAL #1

WHAT I ATE

CALORIES

TIME OF DAY

HUNGER BEFORE

HUNGER AFTER

STARS: ☐ PROTEIN ☐ FIBER ☐ GOOD FATS ☐ FRUITS/VEGGIES

MEAL #2

WHAT I ATE

CALORIES

TIME OF DAY

HUNGER BEFORE

HUNGER AFTER

STARS: ☐ PROTEIN ☐ FIBER ☐ GOOD FATS ☐ FRUITS/VEGGIES

MEAL #3

WHAT I ATE

CALORIES

TIME OF DAY

HUNGER BEFORE

HUNGER AFTER

STARS: ☐ PROTEIN ☐ FIBER ☐ GOOD FATS ☐ FRUITS/VEGGIES

MEAL #4

WHAT I ATE

CALORIES	TIME OF DAY
HUNGER BEFORE	HUNGER AFTER

STARS: ❑ PROTEIN ❑ FIBER ❑ GOOD FATS ❑ FRUITS/VEGGIES

MEAL #5

WHAT I ATE

CALORIES	TIME OF DAY
HUNGER BEFORE	HUNGER AFTER

STARS: ❑ PROTEIN ❑ FIBER ❑ GOOD FATS ❑ FRUITS/VEGGIES

PHYSICAL ACTIVITY

Activity:
Duration:
Intensity:
Calories Burned:

Activity:
Duration:
Intensity:
Calories Burned:

OTHER NOTES

TOTAL CALORIES FOR THE DAY:

TOTAL STARS FOR THE DAY:

Protein

Fiber

Good Fats

Fruits/Veggies

date:

weight:

MEAL #1

WHAT I ATE

CALORIES

TIME
OF DAY

HUNGER
BEFORE

HUNGER
AFTER

STARS: ☐ PROTEIN ☐ FIBER ☐ GOOD FATS ☐ FRUITS/VEGGIES

MEAL #2

WHAT I ATE

CALORIES

TIME
OF DAY

HUNGER
BEFORE

HUNGER
AFTER

STARS: ☐ PROTEIN ☐ FIBER ☐ GOOD FATS ☐ FRUITS/VEGGIES

MEAL #3

WHAT I ATE

CALORIES

TIME
OF DAY

HUNGER
BEFORE

HUNGER
AFTER

STARS: ☐ PROTEIN ☐ FIBER ☐ GOOD FATS ☐ FRUITS/VEGGIES

MEAL #4

WHAT I ATE

CALORIES	TIME OF DAY
HUNGER BEFORE	HUNGER AFTER

STARS: ☐ PROTEIN ☐ FIBER ☐ GOOD FATS ☐ FRUITS/VEGGIES

MEAL #5

WHAT I ATE

CALORIES	TIME OF DAY
HUNGER BEFORE	HUNGER AFTER

STARS: ☐ PROTEIN ☐ FIBER ☐ GOOD FATS ☐ FRUITS/VEGGIES

PHYSICAL ACTIVITY

Activity:
Duration:
Intensity:
Calories Burned:

Activity:
Duration:
Intensity:
Calories Burned:

OTHER NOTES

TOTAL CALORIES FOR THE DAY:

TOTAL STARS FOR THE DAY:

Protein
☐ ☐ ☐ ☐ ☐

Fiber
☐ ☐ ☐ ☐ ☐

Good Fats
☐ ☐ ☐ ☐ ☐

Fruits/Veggies
☐ ☐ ☐ ☐ ☐

date:

weight:

MEAL #1

WHAT I ATE

| CALORIES | TIME OF DAY |

| HUNGER BEFORE | HUNGER AFTER |

STARS: ☐ PROTEIN ☐ FIBER ☐ GOOD FATS ☐ FRUITS/VEGGIES

MEAL #2

WHAT I ATE

| CALORIES | TIME OF DAY |

| HUNGER BEFORE | HUNGER AFTER |

STARS: ☐ PROTEIN ☐ FIBER ☐ GOOD FATS ☐ FRUITS/VEGGIES

MEAL #3

WHAT I ATE

| CALORIES | TIME OF DAY |

| HUNGER BEFORE | HUNGER AFTER |

STARS: ☐ PROTEIN ☐ FIBER ☐ GOOD FATS ☐ FRUITS/VEGGIES

MEAL #4

WHAT I ATE

CALORIES	TIME OF DAY

HUNGER BEFORE	HUNGER AFTER

STARS: ☐ PROTEIN ☐ FIBER ☐ GOOD FATS ☐ FRUITS/VEGGIES

MEAL #5

WHAT I ATE

CALORIES	TIME OF DAY

HUNGER BEFORE	HUNGER AFTER

STARS: ☐ PROTEIN ☐ FIBER ☐ GOOD FATS ☐ FRUITS/VEGGIES

PHYSICAL ACTIVITY

Activity:
Duration:
Intensity:
Calories Burned:

Activity:
Duration:
Intensity:
Calories Burned:

OTHER NOTES

TOTAL CALORIES FOR THE DAY:

TOTAL STARS FOR THE DAY:

Protein
☐ ☐ ☐ ☐ ☐

Fiber
☐ ☐ ☐ ☐ ☐

Good Fats
☐ ☐ ☐ ☐ ☐

Fruits/Veggies
☐ ☐ ☐ ☐ ☐

date:

weight:

MEAL #1

WHAT I ATE

| CALORIES | TIME OF DAY |
| HUNGER BEFORE | HUNGER AFTER |

STARS: ☐ PROTEIN ☐ FIBER ☐ GOOD FATS ☐ FRUITS/VEGGIES

MEAL #2

WHAT I ATE

| CALORIES | TIME OF DAY |
| HUNGER BEFORE | HUNGER AFTER |

STARS: ☐ PROTEIN ☐ FIBER ☐ GOOD FATS ☐ FRUITS/VEGGIES

MEAL #3

WHAT I ATE

| CALORIES | TIME OF DAY |
| HUNGER BEFORE | HUNGER AFTER |

STARS: ☐ PROTEIN ☐ FIBER ☐ GOOD FATS ☐ FRUITS/VEGGIES

MEAL #4

WHAT I ATE

CALORIES	TIME OF DAY

HUNGER BEFORE	HUNGER AFTER

STARS: ☐ PROTEIN ☐ FIBER ☐ GOOD FATS ☐ FRUITS/VEGGIES

MEAL #5

WHAT I ATE

CALORIES	TIME OF DAY

HUNGER BEFORE	HUNGER AFTER

STARS: ☐ PROTEIN ☐ FIBER ☐ GOOD FATS ☐ FRUITS/VEGGIES

PHYSICAL ACTIVITY

Activity:
Duration:
Intensity:
Calories Burned:

Activity:
Duration:
Intensity:
Calories Burned:

OTHER NOTES

TOTAL CALORIES FOR THE DAY:

TOTAL STARS FOR THE DAY:

Protein

Fiber

Good Fats

Fruits/Veggies

date:

weight:

MEAL #1

WHAT I ATE

CALORIES

TIME OF DAY

HUNGER BEFORE

HUNGER AFTER

STARS: ☐ PROTEIN ☐ FIBER ☐ GOOD FATS ☐ FRUITS/VEGGIES

MEAL #2

WHAT I ATE

CALORIES

TIME OF DAY

HUNGER BEFORE

HUNGER AFTER

STARS: ☐ PROTEIN ☐ FIBER ☐ GOOD FATS ☐ FRUITS/VEGGIES

MEAL #3

WHAT I ATE

CALORIES

TIME OF DAY

HUNGER BEFORE

HUNGER AFTER

STARS: ☐ PROTEIN ☐ FIBER ☐ GOOD FATS ☐ FRUITS/VEGGIES

MEAL #4

WHAT I ATE

CALORIES

TIME OF DAY

HUNGER BEFORE

HUNGER AFTER

STARS: ☐ PROTEIN ☐ FIBER ☐ GOOD FATS ☐ FRUITS/VEGGIES

MEAL #5

WHAT I ATE

CALORIES

TIME OF DAY

HUNGER BEFORE

HUNGER AFTER

STARS: ☐ PROTEIN ☐ FIBER ☐ GOOD FATS ☐ FRUITS/VEGGIES

PHYSICAL ACTIVITY

Activity:
Duration:
Intensity:
Calories Burned:

Activity:
Duration:
Intensity:
Calories Burned:

OTHER NOTES

TOTAL CALORIES FOR THE DAY:

TOTAL STARS FOR THE DAY:

Protein

☐ ☐ ☐ ☐ ☐

Fiber

☐ ☐ ☐ ☐ ☐

Good Fats

☐ ☐ ☐ ☐ ☐

Fruits/Veggies

☐ ☐ ☐ ☐ ☐

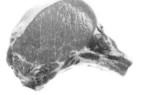

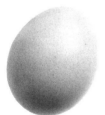

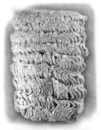

List of
FOODS

FOOD	STANDARD SERVING SIZE	CALORIES
MEAT		
Bacon	1 slice	50
Ground beef, 90% lean	½ cup (about 3 oz)	190
Ham, deli, lean	3 oz	90
Hamburger patty, extra-lean	1 (3 oz)	130
Hamburger patty, 90% lean	1 (3 oz)	180
Pork chop	1 (3 oz)	200
Prosciutto	2 slices	60
Roast beef	2 oz	120
Sausage, smoked, low-fat	½ cup sliced (about 3 oz)	90
Steak, London broil, lean, grilled	3 oz	170
POULTRY AND EGGS		
Chicken breast, grilled	3 oz	140
Chicken drumstick or thigh, without skin	1	110
Egg	1 large	80
Egg whites	2	30
Turkey breast, deli	2 oz	60

FOOD	STANDARD SERVING SIZE	CALORIES
Turkey breast, roast	2 oz (2 small slices)	80
Turkey, ground, 92% or 93% lean	2 oz	80
FISH AND SEAFOOD		
Cod	4 oz raw	120
Crab cake	1 mini (½ oz)	30
Salmon burger	4 oz raw	240
Salmon, grilled	4 oz raw	240
Salmon, smoked	3 oz	130
Sushi—California roll	4 pieces	150
Sushi—spicy tuna roll	4 pieces	140
Tilapia	3 oz (cooked)	110
Tuna, light	3 oz	90
Tuna salad, reduced fat	½ cup	130
Scallop wrapped in bacon	1 scallop	50
Shrimp cocktail	3 shrimp, ½ cup cocktail sauce	50
Shrimp, frozen	4 oz	120
Shrimp, large, brushed with olive oil and grilled	6 shrimp, 2 tsp olive oil	140
BEANS & MEATLESS PROTEINS		
Black beans	½ cup	70
Black beans, refried	½ cup	110
Cannellini beans	½ cup	110
Chickpeas, canned	½ cup	140
Falafel balls	2	110
Hummus	½ cup	210
Lentils	½ cup	120
Soybeans (edamame)	½ cup	100
Stuffed grape leaves	3	120
Three-bean salad	½ cup	90

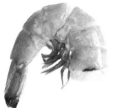

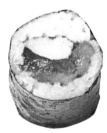

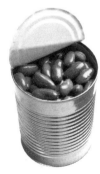

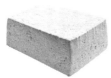

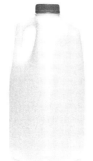

FOOD	STANDARD SERVING SIZE	CALORIES
Tofu, extra-firm	½ cup (4 oz)	100
Tofu, silken	3 oz	50
Soy burger, Boca All American	1 patty	120
Vegetarian chili, canned	½ cup	90
DAIRY & DAIRY ALTERNATIVES		
American cheese	2 slices	140
Asiago cheese	1 oz	110
Blue cheese, crumbled	2 Tbsp	60
Cheddar cheese, reduced fat, grated	2 Tbsp	50
Cottage cheese, 1%	½ cup	80
Cream Cheese, Philadelphia ⅓ Less Fat	2 Tbsp	70
Feta cheese, reduced fat	¼ cup	70
Goat cheese	1 oz (2 Tbsp)	80
Greek Yogurt, Chobani Lowfat Plain	6 oz	130
Mexican cheese (queso blanco), reduced fat, shredded	2 Tbsp	40
Milk, low-fat or fat-free	1 cup	100
Monterey Jack cheese, shredded	2 Tbsp	50
Monterey Pepper Jack cheese, Cabot 50% Reduced Fat	1 oz	70
Mozzarella, part-skim, grated	¼ cup	80
Parmesan cheese, grated	2 Tbsp	40
Parmigiano-Reggiano cheese, grated	½ oz	60
Provolone cheese	Thin slice (½ oz)	50
Rice milk	1 cup	120
Ricotta cheese, part-skim	¼ cup	70
Soy milk	1 cup	110
Swiss cheese, Alpine Lace	Thin slice (½ oz)	50
Whipped cream, fresh	¼ cup	100

FOOD	STANDARD SERVING SIZE	CALORIES
Yogurt, Dannon Light & Fit	6 oz	80
Yogurt, plain low-fat or nonfat	¾ cup	120
BREADS		
Bagel, Pepperidge Farm Brown Sugar Cinnamon Mini	1	120
Bagel, plain	1 (4")	290
Bagel, plain, with cream cheese	1 (4") bagel, 2 Tbsp cream cheese	350
Bagel, whole wheat, hollowed out	1 (4") bagel	230
Bread, 100% whole wheat	2 slices	140
Bread, crusty Italian	1 medium slice (2 oz)	150
Bread, garlic	1 medium slice (2 oz)	210
Bread, rye	1 slice	80
Bread, white	2 slices	130
Bread, whole grain	1 slice	70
Croutons, plain	2 Tbsp	15
Croutons, seasoned	2 Tbsp	25
English muffin	1	130
Hamburger bun	1	120
Hot dog bun	1	120
Pita	1 (6½")	170
Pita Pocket Bread, WeightWatchers 100% Whole Wheat	1	100
Roll, dinner	1 small	80
Sandwich Thins, Arnold Multi-Grain	1 piece	100
Toast, whole wheat, with butter	1 slice	100
Toast, whole wheat, with jam	1 slice	90
Tortilla chips, baked	1 oz	120
Tortilla, corn	1 (6")	60
Tortilla, flour	1 (6")	140

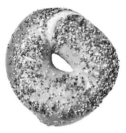

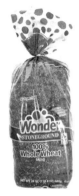

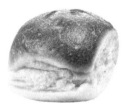

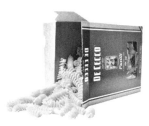

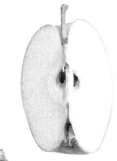

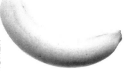

FOOD	STANDARD SERVING SIZE	CALORIES
Tortilla, flour	1 (10")	220
Tortilla, whole wheat	2 oz	120
CEREALS		
Cheerios	1 cup	100
Cornflakes	1 cup	100
Granola, low-fat	½ cup	190
Muesli, five-grain	½ cup	140
Oatmeal	½ cup	80
Wheat germ	1 Tbsp	30
PASTA AND GRAINS (CALORIES FOR COOKED PORTION)		
Barley	½ cup	100
Pasta	1 cup	220
Spaghetti, whole wheat	1 cup	170
Soba noodles	1 cup	110
Tortellini salad	1/4 cup	100
Rice, brown	1/2 cup	110
Rice, fried	1/2 cup	200
Rice pilaf	1/2 cup	140
Rice, white	½ cup	100
FRUITS		
Apple	1 medium	100
Applesauce, unsweetened	½ cup	50
Apricots, dried	4 whole or 8 halves	70
Banana	1 medium	110
Berries, Cascadian Farm Harvest	½ cup	30
Blackberries, frozen	½ cup	50
Blueberries	½ cup	40
Cantaloupe, cubed	½ cup	25

FOOD	STANDARD SERVING SIZE	CALORIES
Cherries, dried	2 Tbsp	60
Cherries, fresh	½ cup	50
Cranberries, dried	2 Tbsp	50
Fruit, dried and chopped (Sun-Maid)	¼ cup	120
Fruit salad	½ cup	50
Grapefruit	½ medium	50
Grapes, seedless	½ cup	60
Honeydew, cubed	½ cup	30
Kiwifruit	1 medium	50
Mango, sliced	½ cup	50
Orange	1 medium	70
Peach	1 medium	60
Peaches, canned in juice, drained	½ cup	55
Pear	1 medium	100
Pear, canned in juice	½ cup	40
Pineapple, canned in juice	½ cup	50
Raisins	2 Tbsp	50
Raspberries	½ cup	30
Strawberries	½ cup	30
Watermelon	½ cup	25
VEGETABLES		
Alfalfa sprouts	½ cup	5
Asparagus	5 spears	20
Beets	2 medium	40
Broccoli, cooked	½ cup	30
Broccoli, frozen	½ cup	20
Broccoli, raw	½ cup	10
Carrot sticks	½ cup	25
Carrots, baby	10	40
Carrots, cooked	½ cup	30

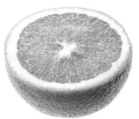

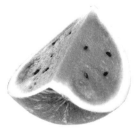

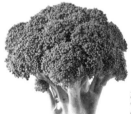

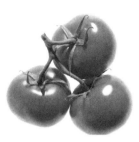
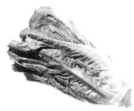
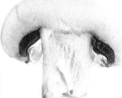

FOOD	STANDARD SERVING SIZE	CALORIES
Celery	½ cup	10
Cole slaw	¼ cup	50
Collard greens	2 cups	20
Corn on the cob	1 medium	80
Cucumber, sliced	½ cup	10
Cucumber salad, marinated	½ cup	25
Green beans, steamed	1 cup	40
Lettuce, mixed greens	1 cup	10
Mixed veggies, frozen	1 cup	40
Mushroom, portobello	1 slice	20
Mushrooms, raw, sliced	½ cup	10
Onion, green, sliced	2 Tbsp	5
Onion, red, sliced	1 slice	10
Pepper, bell, green	1 medium	20
Pepper, bell, red	1 medium	40
Peppers and onions, grilled	½ cup	90
Peppers, roasted	¼ cup	20
Potato, baked	1 medium	160
Potato salad	¼ cup	80
Potatoes, roasted	½ cup	90
Sweet potato	1 medium	100
Spinach, raw or baby	1 cup	10
Tomato	2 slices	10
Tomato	1 medium	20
Tomatoes, cherry	10	30
Water chestnuts	¼ cup	30
Zucchini	¼ cup	5
FATS		
Avocado	¼ cup	60
Butter	1 tsp	30

FOOD	STANDARD SERVING SIZE	CALORIES
Guacamole	1 Tbsp	20
Olive oil	1 tsp	40
Olive oil + red wine vinegar	1 tsp oil, ½ tsp vinegar	40
Olive oil + balsamic vinegar	2 tsp oil, 1 Tbsp vinegar	90
Olive oil + lemon juice	2 tsp oil, 2 tsp lemon juice	80
Olives, sliced	5	50
Sesame oil	1 tsp	40
CONDIMENTS AND SAUCES		
Broth, chicken, low-sodium	1 cup	40
Chutney	1 Tbsp	30
Duck sauce	1 Tbsp	20
Gravy, turkey	2 Tbsp	15
Honey	1 Tbsp	60
Jam, all fruit strawberry	2 tsp	20
Ketchup	1 Tbsp	15
Mayonnaise, light	1 Tbsp	50
Miracle Whip Light	1 Tbsp	40
Mustard, deli	1 tsp	5
Mustard, Dijon	1 tsp	5
Mustard, honey	1 tsp	10
Pasta sauce	⅓ cup	50
Peanut sauce	2 Tbsp	90
Pesto	1 Tbsp	80
Pickles, bread and butter	2 Tbsp	15
Pickle slices	2	0
Salad dressing, Caesar, light	2 Tbsp	30
Salad dressing, Ken's Lite Accents Raspberry Walnut Vinaigrette	10 sprays	15

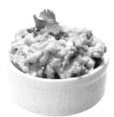

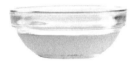

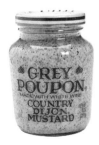

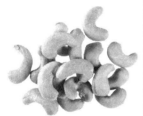

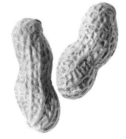

FOOD	STANDARD SERVING SIZE	CALORIES
Salad dressing, Newman's Own Lighten Up Italian Dressing	2 Tbsp	60
Salad dressing, ranch, fat-free	2 Tbsp	40
Salad dressing spray	10 sprays	10
Salsa	¼ cup	20
Soy sauce, low-sodium	1 tsp	5
Sugar, brown	2 tsp	30
Sugar, white	2 tsp	30
Syrup, chocolate	1 Tbsp	60
Syrup, maple	1 Tbsp	50
Tahini	1 Tbsp	50
Teriyaki sauce, low-sodium	2 Tbsp	30
Vinegar, balsamic	1 Tbsp	10
Vinegar, red wine	1 tsp	0
NUTS		
Almond butter	1 Tbsp	100
Almonds, sliced	2 Tbsp	70
Almonds, whole roasted	10	80
Cashews, unsalted	2 Tbsp	100
Coconut, shredded	1 Tbsp	30
Peanut butter	1 Tbsp	90
Peanuts	2 Tbsp	100
Pecans, chopped	2 Tbsp	90
Pine nuts	1 Tbsp	60
Pistachios, chopped	2 Tbsp	90
Sunflower seed kernels, unsalted	1 Tbsp	50
Trail mix	¼ cup	170
Walnut halves	2 Tbsp	80
Walnuts, chopped	2 Tbsp	100

FOOD	STANDARD SERVING SIZE	CALORIES
CAKES, COOKIES, CHIPS, CRACKERS, & CANDY		
Angel food cake	1 slice	70
Apple pie	1 slice (⅛ pie)	300
Cheesecake	1 slice (2½ oz)	260
Chocolate layer cake	4 bites (about 1 oz)	100
Chocolate mousse cake	3 oz (about ⅔ slice)	330
Pound cake	2 oz	220
Mini corn muffin	1 oz	90
Yellow cupcake with chocolate frosting	Small (2.5 oz) cupcake, 2 Tbsp frosting	380
Doritos	1 oz	150
Fritos	1 oz	160
Lay's Potato Chips	1 oz	150
Rice cakes	2	70
Dark chocolate candy bar	2.6 oz	390
Mini chocolate chips	2 Tbsp	100
Mini peanut butter cups	5 pieces	180
Candy-coated peanuts	20 pieces	210
M&Ms	30 pieces	100
Triscuits	6 crackers	120
RyKrisp	2 crackers	60
Wheat Thins	16 crackers	150
Biscotti	2 biscotti	180
Caramel cakes	4 cakes	200
Chocolate chip cookies	2 cookies	110
Oatmeal cookies	2 cookies	90
Fortune cookie	1 cookie	30
Graham cracker squares	2 squares	60

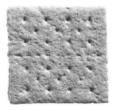

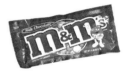

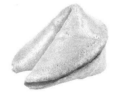

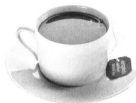

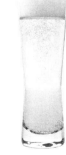

FOOD	STANDARD SERVING SIZE	CALORIES
FROZEN DESSERTS		
Chocolate pudding, fat-free	1 (3½ oz) mini cup	90
Cool Whip, Light	2 Tbsp	20
Frozen yogurt	½ cup	110
Fudge Bar, Skinny Cow	1 bar	100
Ice cream, vanilla	½ cup	140
Pudding, sugar-free	1 (3½ oz) mini cup	25
Sorbet	½ cup	80
BEVERAGES		
Beer, light	12 oz	100
Bloody Mary	6 oz	120
Cappuccino (8 oz skim milk)	16 oz	80
Champagne	5 oz	110
Cocoa, hot, sugar-free	1 packet	50
Coffee with half-and-half	1 cup, 1 Tbsp half-and-half	20
Cosmopolitan	5 oz	250
Gatorade	1 cup	60
Grapefruit juice	1 cup	90
Iced tea, sweet	1 cup	60
Lemonade + unsweetened iced tea, ½ cup each	1 cup	50
Martini	3 oz	170
Orange juice	1 cup	110
Pomegranate-cranberry juice drink + seltzer, ½ cup each	1 cup	50
Sangria + seltzer, ½ cup each	1 cup	80
V8, low-sodium	1 cup	50
Wine, red	5 oz	120
Wine, white	5 oz	120

List of ACTIVITIES

Ways to Burn 400 Calories

ACTIVITY	TIME NEEDED TO BURN 400 CALORIES*
Running a 10-minute mile (6 miles per hour)	35 minutes
Working out on a stair-climbing machine	39 minutes
Mountain biking	42 minutes
Playing singles tennis	44 minutes
Swimming laps (moderate)	50 minutes
Taking an aerobics class (moderate)	54 minutes
Riding a bike at a leisurely pace	59 minutes
Shoveling snow	59 minutes
Rearranging furniture	59 minutes
Ice skating for fun	1 hour and 4 minutes
Mowing the lawn	1 hour and 4 minutes
Walking for exercise (4.0 miles per hour)	1 hour and 11 minutes
Kayaking	1 hour and 11 minutes
Weeding the garden	1 hour and 18 minutes
Dancing in your living room	1 hour and 18 minutes
Playing outside with kids (moderate)	1 hour and 28 minutes

ACTIVITY	TIME NEEDED TO BURN 400 CALORIES*
Walking for exercise (3.5 miles per hour)	1 hour and 33 minutes
Vacuuming	1 hour and 41 minutes
Strength training/ weight lifting (moderate)	1 hour and 58 minutes
Practicing hatha yoga	2 hours and 21 minutes
Watching TV	5 hours and 53 minutes
Sleeping	6 hours and 32 minutes

*Calculations based on a 150-pound person

Source: Ainsworth BE. *The Compendium of Physical Activities Tracking Guide.* Prevention Research Center, Norman J. Arnold School of Public Health, University of South Carolina. 2002, January.